The Human Kind

A Doctor's Stories From the Heart of Medicine

DR PETER DORWARD

GREEN TREE

LONDON • OXFORD • NEW YORK • NEW DELHI • SYDNEY

Moving, compassionate and beautifully written – this book illuminates general practice the way Henry Marsh has illuminated neurosurgery. Dorward's stories from his practice are subtle, eloquent and told with great integrity. He doesn't shy away from confronting some of the most difficult challenges in medicine: refractory pain, chronic fatigue syndrome, maintaining empathy, complex functional illness. But he carries the reader through with verve, imagination, and great humanity. I loved it.

Gavin Francis, author of the *Sunday Times* bestseller *Adventures in Human Being*.

www.gavinfrancis.com
@gavinfranc

For Morrison Dorward, 1928–2017

*Ple... ...doctor.
Howe... ...re that the
identiti... ...ne cases the
stories... ...rent times.
...ted.*

BLOOMSBURY, GREEN TREE and the GREEN TREE logo are trademarks
of Bloomsbury Publishing Plc

First published in Great Britain 2018
This paperback edition published in 2019

Copyright © Peter Dorward, 2018

Peter Dorward has asserted his right under the Copyright, Designs and
Patents Act, 1988, to be identified as Author of this work

A catalogue record for this book is available from the British Library

Library of Congress Cataloguing-in-Publication data has been applied for

ISBN: PB: 9781472943941; eBook: 9781472943910; epdf: 9781472943927

2 4 6 8 10 9 7 5 3 1

Typeset in Fournier MT Std by Deanta Global Publishing Services, Chennai, India
Printed and bound by CPI Group (UK) Ltd, Croydon, CR0 4YY

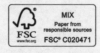

To find out more about our authors and books visit www.bloomsbury.com
and sign up for our newsletters

CONTENTS

Narcotics cannot still the tooth that nibbles at the soul ...

Emily Dickinson

Introduction

A Private Garden

To never have to feel as tired as this again...
To never have to feel so wretched...
Oh...

A young doctor sits with his head in his hands at a trestle table in the staff canteen of a district general hospital in Northern England. He wears an old-style white coat: stained and crumpled with use, a stethoscope in one pocket, a book jammed in the other, two bleeps in the breast pocket, one marked with peeling red duct tape. It's half past seven in the morning and still dark outside. It's 1989, and it's been raining for years. He has a mug of tea sitting cupped between his hands, getting cold now. Work started the previous morning at half past eight. He will get home again at eight that evening.

He's thinking: *I never want to have to feel this tired again. I never want to feel this wretched.*

'Bad night?'

Someone sits opposite him.

'Shelley. Hi.'

He is unenthusiastic to see her. Shelley is a year or two older than he is. She's from *Zim*, Rhodesia, as she sometimes says, by mistake. She's thin, has cropped dark hair, intense blue eyes. She is remarkably impervious to strain. She, too, has been up all night: she, if anything, has had it harder, because it's Sunday morning, and there is no place harder than the casualty department of that hospital, in that town, on a Saturday night. But Shelley is fresh and manicured: clean white coat, clean blouse. Somewhere, somehow, she has found a place to shower. She doesn't have that up-all-night-in-casualty smell on her – that special alcohol/sick/blood combo we all *so* know – and her eye make-up is this morning's, not last night's, you can tell. She has brought two cups of tea, one for herself, the other fresh, hot, for him. Tiny acts of kindness go far in this bleak world. He makes an effort to wake.

'You look terrible.'

'Thanks!'

'How did Mr Foster do?'

'Died.'

'Bad?'

'Not great…'

Then, from nowhere, a great surge of emotion, a welling up, intimations of a sob. A bellyful of something hot, rising in his throat, threatens to explode. He swallows hard: *Down! Keep these rebel feelings DOWN!*

Shelley, who was standing, about to leave, sits down again, waits a mo.

'Actually, really … really crap…'

Sob. Swallow.

12 hours earlier.

Feeling great – *Ward under control, set fair for a quiet-ish night, lots of energy still in the tank, might even get some sleep* – when his bleep goes off. It's Shelley calling from casualty:

'Gerald Foster's back again. Haematemesis. Vitals are stable but he looks a little grey. Bloods are all gone off and he's got a unit of O neg up, but he'll be coming your way.'

Gerald Foster was what might be called a regular. He had been a very serious alcoholic once. Now in his mid-sixties, he has oesophageal varices, a complication of alcoholic liver disease. Blood, unable to make its way through his rock-like liver, backs up in other places: in his case, in the blood vessels around the bottom of his oesophagus. These varices sit around the mouth of the stomach like over-ripe grapes, ready to rupture. When they do, he bleeds, and when he does, he vomits. Haematemesis.

Young Doctor makes his way down to casualty at a brisk walk. The walls are painted pale green. The corridors are cluttered with patient trolleys and old-style metal drip stands. A porter with a spiderweb tattoo on his neck stands by a lift, surreptitiously smoking. Remember: it's 1989.

'Ho, Pete!' says the porter.

'Spider!' says Pete, who doesn't much like to be called *Pete*, but nonetheless likes the human contact, and wishes he could have a cigarette too.

Mr Foster is sitting up in resus., grey indeed, drinking tea and eating a slice of toast. Emaciated man, stick limbs, big belly, white wispy hair, a touch of jaundice, fresh NHS issue paper gown protecting his modesty, his clothes in plastic bags by the trolley; there is blood caked still on his chin and chest.

'Good evening, Mr Foster.'

'Who are you?'

Mr Foster crunches on a slice of toast. Butter runs down his chin.

'I'm Doctor Dorward. I'm here to check you out...' He feels the man's pulse, by way of getting started, although there's a machine doing all that already. He leans over, then

3

leans back and swallows quickly. Butter, blood, tea, vomit, and Mr Foster is unkempt at the best of times. He leans back in again, checks the man's eyes.

Mr Foster: 'Who are you?'

'Doesn't matter...'

He suffers from Korsakoff's Syndrome, a not-so-rare complication of alcoholic brain disease. It's caused by vitamin deficiency and neglect, easily prevented, impossible to cure. It means that Mr Foster has no short-term memory. He doesn't remember a thing, from one moment to the next. The doctor listens to his chest, puts a hand on the abdomen, feels for the liver, feels for tenderness.

'Gerroff! *Fuckitt!* Who are you? Where am I?'

Mr Foster doesn't remember, from one moment to the next. In his case that's probably just as well. Mr Foster used to be a small-town bank manager. He had had a house in a nice area, a car and two teenage daughters who attended private school, but he lost all of that. Mr Foster had served a short prison sentence in the late seventies for sexual offences against a child. Upon his release, everything was lost: the job, the house, the car, the family. He didn't want them any more in any case. The alcohol was a kind of slow suicide, now half completed.

'Where am I?'

'Doesn't matter...'

A nurse has appeared at the bedside, checking observations, marking them on a chart hanging at the bottom of the trolley.

'He shouldn't be eating! He should be nil-by-mouth.'

'No one told *us!*' she says, back now turned, leaving.

This hospital, with its casualty department, is due to close in a year. A few miles down the motorway a new one has been built – half the services have been transferred across already. A new building, all steel and glass. There, the nursing staff are young, confident and enthusiastic. There is a central nursing bay for ease of communication. They have an up-to-date telephone system, innovative new computer terminals and training programmes on how to use them. There, the nursing staff wouldn't have to be *told* that tea and toast were wrong for Mr Foster, they would just *know*. The new hospital has drained the life from this, the old. This hospital is blighted.

'They're giving him tea and toast!' says the young doctor, gearing up for a *huge moan* about the nursing staff.

'They're just being kind,' says Shelley, signing off on one set of notes, picking up another from the pile.

'They're meant to be bloody *nurses!*'

'They *are* nurses. They're just trying to be kind,' she says, leaving.

Shelley is not very popular. Sanctimonious. And white Rhodesians are considered fair game. Although right on the bottom rung of the hierarchy, as a doctor, she is in a different league. She has worked in the townships: she seems to have seen *everything*. She is unfazed by stabbings. Gunshot wounds are *nothing* to Shelley. There is something of the missionary about her. She wears a cross on a chain. She is aloof. She never joins in, she never complains, never bitches about the nurses. She's always talking about her boyfriend, Wilhelm, whom she's marrying in the summer: a great white wedding in South Africa, if the summer ever comes. She makes people feel judged. At least that's what people accuse her of, unkindly, as they mimic her accent behind her back.

Mr Foster vomited again almost as soon as he got up to the ward. Usually he just settles down. Usually it's just a question of replacing blood and fluids, maybe a little morphine for his blood pressure and a sedative for general distress – his, and the ward's. On the ward, he'll be shouting out, again and again, all night 'Where the hell am I?' while the other patients complain and the nursing staff bite their lips and ignore him. The young doctor cross-matches him for 4 units of blood, puts in a bigger central intravenous line for quick resuscitation, and transfers him to intensive care.

Intensive care is not at all what you might think. It isn't as if there is a hierarchy of intensivists, anaesthetists, surgeons, pharmacologists, a team of highly trained nurses, skilled and ready to take over. It's 1989, and the hospital is blighted. Intensive care is a bay, a biggish room, at the end of one of the wards. There *is* a consultant on duty, but he is covering the other hospital, he's busy, and there is some political aspect to the consultant rota which the doctor doesn't fully understand. For whatever reason, when he has called for help before, he has been met with a frosty response and gently chastised by his *own* boss the following morning.

But Mr Foster vomits more blood: it's not even clotted now, and his haemoglobin has come back at 5.2. Normal would be 13. He's lost more than half his blood volume. He calls the duty consultant. The duty consultant asks whether the surgeons have been consulted.

'Surgeons deal with out-of-hours upper gastrointestinal bleeding. Have you spoken with them?'

'Where am I?' wails the grey man from the bed opposite, then vomits some more.

The surgeon points out that there is nothing that they will do: the patient needs adequate fluid resuscitation. 'Who do you think I am? The Wizard of Oz? Stabilise him. Call us in the morning.'

There's two units of whole blood available now though, and that goes up, goes through, and Mr Foster's blood pressure seems to stabilise.

There's other stuff to be done in the hospital, there always is. A young man is admitted with an acute MI. He's stable enough, but needs active treatment. Heart attacks have recently been re-branded. The possibility of 'clot-busting' drugs has just been developed: it's no longer a question of giving morphine and putting the patient in a bed by a defibrillator and letting them take their chances. There are doses to be figured out, unfamiliar new drugs to be administered, drop by drop. There is a run of old men with pneumonia, and a teenager with asthma. It's all routine, it's not really *busy* as such, but it's late by the time the doctor gets back to his patient in intensive care.

The charge nurse in the intensive care unit has years of experience. Stanley is the kind of stable, benign, coping night-time presence that junior doctors yearn for. Last really good nurse left hanging on: the rest have left. *The last leaf on the tree.* But Stanley looks worried as hell. 'We're not really keeping up with Mr Foster. He's had all four units, but he's not really settling.'

He seems to be asleep. Still grey-white, blue tinged lips, but sleeping at least.

'At least he's stopped vomiting…'

The last of the colour then drains from Mr Foster's face. 'Whoops!' says Stanley. Mr Foster vomits again, fresh unclotted blood, the contents, at least, of those four units just squeezed in.

Stanley takes the head end with a sucker: clears the airway, but there's always more to come. The suction bottle, already half full before this, needs changing.

It's 5 a.m. It's the dead time of night. The junior doctor is back on the phone to the duty surgeon.

'There's nothing we can do until he's stable. Have you passed a Sengstaken tube?'

A Sengstaken tube is a kind of inflatable plastic tube thing that you would put down a person's throat in 1989 if you wanted to stop bleeding from the oesophagus. This hadn't actually occurred to the junior doctor as an option, although Stanley already has one ready. The junior doctor has as little expertise in their use as you do. Mr Foster is well awake now and is thrashing around like a hooked fish. Stanley suggests some morphine, and some more, and then some Valium, and Mr Foster seems more settled. But his breathing is rasping now, rattling, intermittent. His colour is awful.

'Have you passed one of these before, Pete?' asks Stanley, wiping down the Sengstaken tube, but at that moment, Mr Foster stops breathing, and the trace on his ECG goes flat.

The junior doctor immediately starts chest compressions, but Stanley puts a hand on his shoulder and says, 'Pete!'

'What?'

'Mr Foster is at the bottom of a huge slope. If you start his heart again, which you won't, he will still have no blood. And if you give him 10 units of blood, which we don't have, he'll still have a massive bleeding point in his oesophagus. And if we sort that out, he'll still have no memory, he still won't know who he is. And if you miraculously fix *that*, he'll still want to be dead anyway. Think we should mebbe stop?'

Not really Stanley's call, and a bit long-winded perhaps, but these were his words: this is the speech that the doctor remembers, even now, 30 years later. He remembers that Stanley was twice his age, had ten times his experience, had a great heart, and knew a broken doctor when he saw one.

The surgeon ambles in at last, laughs like a drain, and says, 'Left this one a bit late, haven't you?'

Stanley keeps his hand on the doctor's shoulder and says, 'I'll clear up, Pete. You get yourself a cup of tea.'

———

To never have to feel as tired as this again…
To never have to feel so wretched…

With enormous effort, the junior doctor pulls himself together. He's 26. It absolutely doesn't do to sob and wail and say 'I just want to go home', even in front of Shelley – even though she now seems the most compassionate, mature, discreet and reliable person in the world, who has just brought him some toast as well, to match the hot tea. That second little act of kindness, at the end of a grim night, it melts the soul.

'It was … really … crap.'

'One for the private garden?'

What private garden?

'We all have one,' says Shelley, tapping the side of her head. 'A private place. The garden of remembrance. Where we remember all the things that go wrong. The heartbreaks? We all have them, or at least we should. All those stories that would break us if we thought about them all the time, but can't let go of all the same? The garden of remembrance. You can go there from time to time.'

She sips her tea. So does he. His bleep goes off. Medical ward.

It can probably wait.

It probably can't.

'You can go there from time to time. *You* clearly need to. Not too often though.' She looks at her watch, then smiles, winks, leaves.

———

A private garden.

A place for memories, and the ghosts of memories. Those memories that broke your heart, those that changed you, the ones that made you reconsider everything, again, from the very beginning – the ones that make you start over, the ones that make you who you are.

My garden is now better stocked, more mature, better tended: far more peaceful than it was in 1989. Much visited. A place for memories, half-memories, and ghosts. Was I really quite as *alone* as I remember those events back then? *That* wouldn't happen now, I hope.

But I can remember Mr Foster, and his wispy white hair, and his toast with butter. I remember Shelley, that's for sure, and her words. I remember feeling so alone, not knowing what I *should* have done.

———

When I think about medicine, I think about people. Their voices, the words they used, their bodies and their faces, their relationships, the way they made me *feel* – when I think or talk about medicine, these flicker through my memory.

The facts of a case: the numbers, the signs, the science, the rarity, the amazing, miraculous cures, the smart diagnoses and the cleverness of the person that spotted them – these things are of great but passing interest. But what changes us – or me, at any rate – are the people attached to those facts. Those whom we accompany, walk with for a while through a part of their lives, sometimes even to the very edges of their lives. Those people whom we influence, and most influence us.

To fix a person who is sick, the facts of their damaged body, the nature and origin of the harm, and the skill to fix it must be clear in front of us. But unless we know the purpose of that body – what it means to itself, how it functions in the world, what about it matters to its owner, or whether it matters at all – there still won't be any hope for remedy for the person, however we try.

No accumulation of facts about a body will tell us why the person it contains is sometimes kind to it, and sometimes so hateful. No accumulation of fact will tell us when we should try *really hard*, or sometimes *not so hard*, or *not at all*, or whether we should treat every single human body in the world *just the same*. There's no clear rule or test that might safely help us determine that. No accumulation of knowledge or facts about the world will give us answers to questions about how we should behave in it.

I think that our culture is, by and large, expert in the *facts*, the *science* of how the world works: so expert, in fact, that our knowledge and skill blinds us to other things. We use the tools of science to try to solve problems intractable to them, and we do this in the world of medicine more than in most others. I think that we need to think more clearly about what sorts of problems are solvable by facts and science, and what aren't. I think we need to think more clearly about what tools we might better use instead.

I don't know the answers to these questions. Nonetheless, I would like to make the most modest possible claim: we don't think enough about these things. We'll all get to be patients in the end (some quite soon), so it's urgent. Even though these problems have existed since there have been people to think about them, we still need to think about them more.

———

This is a walk through my garden. It is populated by memories and the ghosts of memories. I have tried to follow the thread of my argument through the voices and stories of people. But these *are* stories: the memories behind them, their first stimulus, has been altered, adapted, re-attributed, shuffled, mixed, changed, until their origins are lost in the mosaic. In those cases where I have used words or a story given to me by a person I can identify, I have asked that person, and I am grateful for their willing consent.

On the other hand, I hope that everyone reading this will recognise in it at least something of their own story. Nothing that I have written about here is very rare, and most of the problems I and my patients struggle with, are common problems: those broken threads of paradox, confusion, suffering, joy, dissonance and incoherence that are woven through the fabric of our experience.

Zennor, August 2017

I Just Want to Help you to Die

I met this man – he was a lovely man – but I wanted nothing more than to help him to die.

The first time I see him, he is accompanied by his daughter. He is a man in his mid-sixties. A short, thin, blocky man in a cigarette-singed Hibs football strip. He jumps to his feet when I call his name and surges ahead of his daughter, a smile on his face, as if he is eager to see me. I know his daughter a bit already. She is the carer for another patient of mine – a young man with very severe multiple sclerosis, who depends on her to an extraordinary degree, not just for his mechanical, physical care, but for the kind of emotional sustenance, the kind of intimacy, a kind of love, which everyone needs but can hardly ever be offered by paid, social services carers. So I already know his daughter to be an extraordinary woman, a devoted, kind person whom I admire, and when I see that it is she who is bringing her father, to see *me*, I am flattered. She wears a worried, slightly apologetic expression on her face, common to the children of ageing parents when those parents start to fail. He looks fearful too, that is obvious enough already, when he follows me into my surgery and sits down.

He has a Starbucks styrene cup in his hand. He flips the cap off and presents me with a puddle of blood streaked with pus and says to me 'Doctor, does that mean what I think it means?' and his daughter, embarrassed, says 'Dad!' but he cuts her off, says 'No, I want tae ken! Does it mean what I think it means?' He smells of smoke. He has nicotine yellowing his right forefinger, and his fingers are clubbed, the tips swollen like drumsticks. His specimen reeks of tar. Blood and tar – it's a smell you come to dread.

'Have you been coughing that up?'

He nods. I nod, holding his gaze. He looks frightened, but he's defiant too. He tells me that he has been coughing this up for months. His daughter says 'Dad…' again, but not admonishing him this time. He tells me that he has lost weight, isn't eating, can't really get his breath, all the time holding my gaze with these frightened, pale blue eyes of his.

'So it's lung cancer, isn't it, Doc?'

I say I don't know, but knowing really, and examine him. There is the smell of smoke, and Brut, which is an aftershave popular among Scottish men during the seventies which has been, I had thought, unavailable for decades. A hint of half metabolised alcohol. Bony ribs, and without the Hibs strip he is emaciated indeed. When I tap his lungs the right base is dull as stone – stony dull, which means that there is fluid in the chest cavity on the right, which might explain in part why he is so breathless. I ask him to take a deep breath and he raises his ribs and his shoulders in a big bold display of sucking in air, which I think is something that men of his generation learned in the army – a kind of gesture of enthusiastic health – but I don't hear much air moving.

I sit again, facing him, take his hands in mine to inspect again these clubbed fingers. That's another bad sign, at least in men his age, with a body as worn as his, with his gurgling cough and his coughing up of blood.

'So?'

I slide off his question. 'I need to do a chest x-ray. There's definitely something not right in your chest, and I'm worried about it. But I need to do a chest x-ray first.'

He looks a little disappointed.

'But you think it's lung cancer?'

Actually I think I *know* it's lung cancer.

'Dad – the doctor needs to do an x-ray first…'

'I want to know!'

'Well…'

'The thing is, Doctor, I *want* it to be…'

'Dad…!'

'… lung cancer…'

Jim Stuart's wife, Margaret Stuart, died about 18 months ago from breast cancer. I knew her only slightly. She was a frail, anxious woman, biologically much older than her 65 years, driven to old age I suspect by her rumbustious, devoted, demanding husband. When, later, I spend time with Jim in his front room, next to the telly I notice a montage of photographs of them together. Taken somewhere abroad (you can tell by the burned red faces of the company), Jim in his Hibs strip surging forward with a grin and a pint of beer and a cig between his fingers, toasting the lens, and behind him, smiling tolerantly with a wee glass of white wine in her hand, Margaret. Since Margaret died, the daughter, Adie, tells me he hasn't really done anything. Never gets out now, never goes to the little patch of green behind his ground floor flat, with its bed of hard pruned roses and the pair of deck chairs, one blown over by the wind, where he and Margaret had once sat out during summer days. He sits on the couch now, drinking beer, watching the football, smoking his Players No6, telling anyone that asks that he's fine, aye, just fine, doing okay, wishing away his days.

I order a chest x-ray. Jim is a little annoyed that I have evaded his question. Adie thanks me, as if what I have done already is the most wonderful thing in the world.

Charged encounters like the one with Jim, although they don't happen every day, happen most weeks. I'm busy, and by late afternoon I have almost forgotten him. But at 5 p.m. I see that I have a note to phone the x-ray technician at the local hospital, and I know, of course, what it is that she has to tell me. She just wants to give me a heads-up. She's sent through the report, but she just wants to let me know. Jim's x-ray, as I knew it would be, is really bad. One lung is almost obscured by fluid, but where you can see behind the whiteout, there is a large, tentacled mass where the lung joins its bronchial tubes, and there are signs of swollen glands around the heart. I call Adie on her mobile.

'Can you bring him back up?'

'Is it what we think it is?'

'Probably.'

I worry about patient confidentiality. Medical confidentiality is not absolute – it's violable in certain dire situations, such as threats of suicide or murder, or in the cases of the mad or wholly incapable, but ordinarily, what a patient tells you, or what you know about your patient, you keep to yourself. Everybody who knows anything at all about the ethics of medicine would agree with this. If you have news for a patient, like the news I have for Jim, you don't break it to his daughter first. On the other hand, something about Jim strikes me as profoundly vulnerable. I need to have this conversation with Jim, urgently, but I need it to be mediated by the presence of his daughter – this warm, big-hearted woman, who I know cares for him, who I know had his interests at heart, who I know would understand the implications of what I was going to say. From everything that I know, I know that it is for the best that I speak with her first. So I make that judgement.

I'm running very late indeed by the time I call them through again. Jim is a little staggery when he stands, and he calls out to me as he crosses the waiting room, in a voice too loud: 'Doctor, a hope you dinnae mind and it's no disrespect, ken, but ah've had a wee drink.' I smile, to say *no, of course I don't mind,* and Jim says, 'Because I know what you're going to say, I know I've got lung cancer,' and a mother who's waiting in the waiting room with her kids looks up sharply and reaches an arm out for the child playing at her feet.

He sits down again, Adie, who has been crying, beside him. He holds me with these milky blue eyes of his, and says, 'So, Doc, what's it to be?' as if he's offering me a drink.

'Well…' I say, finding my ground, framing the thought, choosing my words, already prevaricating. Jim sniffs the air, scenting hesitation.

There's a skill to breaking bad news. It's an art. We try to teach it to students and trainees, but it is a skill that needs practice like any other, and the longer you do it, the better you become, so long as you keep it up and care to invest in it. First, you create a space which isn't a busy, contested, jumbled space. You create time for silence and reflection. You adopt an open, relaxed pose. You wear a face that isn't grim, but serious nonetheless, not tense, but kind, without being cloying. You warn. You say 'we have to have a serious conversation', or something similar, then check what your patient already knows and understands, and get a first intimation of what it is that they want to know, and understand. You then proceed in small steps. 'The x-ray shows some worrying changes…' and wait for a response, and make the next step based on the response to the last. You don't

17

use euphemisms, and you use words like cancer, and die, if they need to be used, but you don't brutalise your patient with these words if they don't want to hear them. Small steps. You check what has been understood. You finish with a plan, which ideally you've put in place before you even see your patient. 'I have a specialist appointment booked for you on Thursday at nine. They'll want to do some scans to confirm the diagnosis and plan your treatment.' Something like that. You check that you have been understood. You say, 'If you have any questions later on, or tomorrow, or whenever, call me. You know where I am.'

'Well,' I say to Jim, adopting an open, relaxed posture, wearing an expression which I hope isn't grim, an expression not too serious, kind, but...

'Just get to it, Doc. *Ah've* no got all day. How long have I got?'

'I think you're probably right. I think you may have cancer in your right lung. There are lots of other things that it could be, but looking at the x-ray I'd be a bit surprised if it turned out to be anything else.'

Adie is looking at her father, glassy blue eyes wide open, a watery smile on her face.

'Aye, I knew that it was cancer. I've known for months. How long have I got?'

He seems entirely unshaken. A little fearful, sure, but no more than before he knew. He's not drunk. Doesn't seem upset or depressed at all. More relieved.

Doctors are asked the question 'how long have I got?' all the time. It's one of our badly answered questions – one to which we almost always avoid a direct response, for good reasons sometimes, but often for bad. People with predictably life limiting illnesses, such as metastatic cancer, or heart failure, will often enter a kind of plateau phase which will last for weeks or months, or even years.

I once looked after an old woman in her nineties who was discharged from hospital with a ruptured heart valve. Eliza had terminal heart failure and was sent home to be 'kept comfortable'. I agreed to visit her, initially every couple of weeks, to help try to manage her drugs – a tricky balance between giving too much diuretic and causing her kidneys to fail, or too little, causing her heart to be overwhelmed and her lungs to fill with fluid. It's a very common medical scenario – this dismal optimal. The patient for whom *best possible* is actually *pretty grim*. The patient for whom any intervention at all just seems to make things worse.

I got to know her well. She told me that, as a 16-year-old, in 1939, she had been admitted to hospital with appendicitis. Back in those kinder days, she had a couple of weeks' convalescence in hospital, where she was looked after by a young house surgeon called Axel, from Hanover. She went a little pink as she confided, eyes twinkling as she told me, and I began to see a little of what Axel must have seen in her. She had never told her family about their meeting, not for any particular reason other than life, and marriage, and children, deaths, joy, sorrow, and all the other things that complicate a long life. But she and Axel had become a little sweet on one another. He loved books, and so did she. In the most tentative way, an agreement had formed between them that they might meet, sometime later, a decent period after she had been discharged home. She had lent him *Gone With the Wind*, which he hadn't got on with, being a medical man, and unromantic, she said, but the need to return it had become a pretext. They never even held hands. Between them was never anything more than the most tentative of understandings, anything else would have been impossible in those days, and wrong. But of course they never did meet, they never could. Nothing happened. He had had to leave – he had to return to Germany. But for some reason, now at the end of her life, she found herself thinking about her young German doctor from time to time, wondering what had become of him. He had been an extraordinarily kind young man. She dreaded to think what might have become of him.

Eliza's terminal illness lasted for almost two and a half years. She was an immensely clever, cultured woman, who had never had the benefit of a proper education. We talked about books. She loved Graham Greene, Somerset Maugham, Anthony Burgess and Lawrence Durrell. Her tastes were exotic. I suggested books to her, which she would download to the tablet her daughters had bought her. She enjoyed *Any Human Heart* by William Boyd, but thought the hero villainous. She was pained by *The Narrow Road to the Deep North* because she had known men who had been enslaved by the Japanese, and I felt an oaf for having recommended it. She died half way through Margaret Atwood's *Robber Bride*, having struggled with it for months. I thought that she was just stuck, but on reflection, I think that it was due to the opiates I had prescribed to control her breathlessness.

I looked after a man once, a retired accountant with an interest in maths. He was dying of prostate cancer, but in his plateau phase. He asked me a few times how long I thought he had, and I told him I didn't know. One of the characteristics of prostate cancer is that the tumour releases a chemical compound into the blood, called Prostate Specific Antigen, or PSA. It forms the basis for how we detect the condition in the first place. His treatment was being monitored with regular tests. One afternoon, a week or two after his latest bloods, he came to see me with a roll of paper under his arm, which he spread out on my desk in front of him. He had plotted against time, on a long sheet of graph paper, all of his PSA results since his diagnosis, several years before. He pointed out to me a long, gently inclining line, with, in recent months, a noticeable upward flick. I gave him his latest blood test, which he carefully plotted on the paper with a fine, sharp, meticulous old mathematician's pencil. He had discerned the deeper pattern of the numbers. 'This is differential calculus,' he explained to me, using a formula to calculate the trend of the upwardly rising line. 'Newton invented it. You can see here,' he said, pointing to a place in the clearly determined, not-so-distant future, 'when the line starts to rise almost vertically'. He looked at me with a little smile, which some people, calm in the face of death, will sometimes wear. 'Asymptotic. A curve that tends to infinity. I think that that's the answer to my question.'

I once looked after a man, a retired ship's engineer, who had terminal bowel cancer with liver metastases. For a long time he used to come to see me at my surgery, but then, as he weakened, growing thinner and more gaunt, struggling more under the burden of his symptoms, I started to visit him at home. He had asked me once how long he had, and I had told him that I didn't know. The first time I visited him at home, he walked with me to the garden gate, and as we chatted, he placed his bony thigh through the gap between the wrought iron, and pushed, testing. He frowned, shrugged his shoulders, smiled and said, 'It's my engine gauge. I'm disappearing. I never used to be able to get my leg this far in.'

When people ask us how they're doing, how long they have, we prevaricate. They find their own answers.

'We don't know…' I say, then correct myself. When I'm under pressure – I've noticed this in myself and dislike it – I substitute 'I' for 'we'. It's a subtle evasion. '*I* don't know. Perhaps with treatment…'

'I don't want any treatment. No more doctors, no scans, no chemo, no operations. I've got lung cancer. I just want to know how long I have, and go home.'

'He hates doctors,' says Adie, shaking her head. 'I had to drag him here. But he likes you. Don't you, Dad?'

'Aye…' says Jim, provisionally.

'You don't want treatment?'

Shakes his head.

'Even if treatment could help you? Even if treatment could prolong your life?'

'I've got lung cancer.'

Adie takes her father's hand.

I have a certain sympathy for Jim's position. I'm no specialist, but a man with his chest x-ray just isn't going to have a curable disease, supposing that the diagnosis is right, and I'm sure that it is. And I have this long-held suspicion, which may be no more than prejudice, that some specialists, the surgeons and oncologists in this case, aren't always terribly good at knowing when the treatments that they offer are futile. Studies suggest that doctors over-estimate the life expectancies of the terminally ill by a factor of five, and the more engaged in active, curative treatment, the more marked this optimistic tendency. Doctors of the heroic mould can seem blind to the *shortness* of people's lives. Not always terribly good at knowing when to stop. Or being able to frame the question in such a way that 'stop' is a possible answer. The short tail ends of people's lives are squandered if they become nothing but patients, being worried by tests which are always inconclusive, by long waits and cruel drugs followed by inevitable deaths. Time wasted. Unlike us generalists, I sometimes think, the surgeon doesn't have to continue to look after his failures. He need never see them.

But no matter how you try to keep it neutral, people are extraordinarily likely to conform to the interests, prejudices and suggestions of those whom they see as their healers. So humility demands I keep my nihilistic thoughts to myself.

'So tell me how long I've got?'

'I don't know. It would surprise me if you were still alive a year from now. I would be surprised if you died within the next month or two.'

'So that's three months then?'

The *first* rule of breaking bad news is, of course, don't think out loud. I'm still not quite sure how I got here, and quite so fast, but I don't say no.

'Can you give me a note then, Doc.'

'A note?'

'Aye. For her.' He says, nodding at Adie, who is looking at her feet, swallowing her tears.

Eh?

'To tell her not to carry on with they toy boys, after I'm deid.'

Eh?

'He's joking.' Says Adie. 'Dad's *joking*.'

I made a deal with Jim. I persuaded him that, if I agreed to certain of his conditions, he would agree to come to see me every two weeks or so, to keep an eye on things. His conditions were, for me, onerous. They were, essentially, absolute passivity. They were: no specialists, no scans, no tests of any kind; to avoid hospital admission no matter what, and probably no drugs. I also wasn't to pester him about smoking any more, and, of course, drinking. In exchange for that, for my agreeing to swallow this huge mass of indigestible uncertainty, he would agree, provisionally, to let me care for him.

He was standing now, trying to look down on me. With me sitting, he was just about able to. He had these milky blue eyes. His hands shook. Adie stood behind him, hands up, anguish and embarrassment mixed on her face.

'OK, Doc?'

Outmanoeuvred, I agreed.

In his book *Being Mortal*, the American surgeon and writer, Atul Gawande, advocates four simple questions that doctors might ask their terminal patients. I admire Gawande, for his humanity and clarity, and the strength and passion of his purpose, and when I read his book, I immediately resolved to change the way in which I speak with the very sick. British doctors like to think that we are way ahead of the US in palliative care, and that, consequently, although he is greatly admired, Gawande hasn't so much to teach us. I think we're just being complacent. I think that in Scotland we probably do palliative care as badly and as well as anywhere. Gawande suggests, and cites compelling research to back him up, that if you can remember to ask four simple questions of the dying, you will contribute to the easing of their suffering. You will reduce their consumption of medical technology, prolong their lives, and, at the end, reduce their need for palliative drugs. Imagine what investment there would be in a drug that achieved this end? What triumph! What celebration!

First of all, you ask: *What do you understand by your illness? Where are you up to with your treatment? What are your expectations?*

You get your patient to set the scene, begin to open a dialogue based on their thoughts, not yours.

You ask: *Given that, what do you want now? What matters to you? What are your priorities? What trade-offs would you make in order to achieve that?*

You ask: *What do you fear? What barriers are there to realising what you want with what remains of your life?*

Then you ask: *What's your bottom line? What would be unacceptable to you? What must we avoid happening, no matter what?*

So you have a conversation, which is based on your patient's knowledge and understanding of their situation, not yours. Your patient's aspirations and fears. You get to know what your patient wants to avoid, at all costs. It seems so absolutely obvious. So extraordinary that we haven't routinely practised this way forever. So unforgivable, in fact, that often we still don't.

I am pleased and relieved when Jim comes back to see me a couple of weeks later. This time he leaves Adie in the waiting room. He stands alone, gives me a little wave and smiles, says chirpily, 'Ten weeks to go, Doc!', walks unassisted down the corridor to my room. He is already diminished though. Less sure of his balance, less sure of himself, and although he smiles at me, defiantly, I can tell that he is more afraid than ever.

He sits down. I sit opposite him.

'So, Jim,' I say, then pause, then ask, 'Where are you up to? What's been happening to you?'

'I wanted to speak to you privately.' He gestures dismissively with his head towards the door. 'Without *her* yapping on.'

Men do this often, I find, even decent men. The more vulnerable they are, the more disparagingly they speak of the women that love them and keep them alive.

'Okay.' We pause for a moment, holding one another's gaze.

'I know what I want.'

'Good,' I say. 'Good.'

'It's not one of thae bucket lists though. I ken whit's coming my way. I know whit's in the post. I'm no off tae Disnae-Land.'

It sounds like a pun, in Scots. I'm pretty sure he intended it.

'But I don't want her knowing, okay?'

'Okay…' I say, more hesitantly.

'Because I'm done with this.'

I nod, not really understanding.

'But I'm not jumping off a bridge.'

'No,' I say understanding.

'And I'm not jumping in front of a bus. That would be, you know…' He nods again at the door. To *her*. In the waiting room. '… upsetting. You know.'

'Sure.' I nod, my heart heavy in my chest.

These conversations happen less frequently than you might think. For all the near consensus among my friends and relatives that getting old, getting sick, dementing, dying, isn't for them (it certainly isn't for me), when it comes down to it, the number of times that I have had patients telling me about their plans, in this matter of fact manner, not intended for effect, neither a performance of grief nor in any sense a 'cry for help', but as a realistic, planned intention, are few. Once or twice. Until I read *Being Mortal*, that is. Until I learned better skills for talking to the dying.

If you talk to depressed people, or even to not depressed people, but to people who are simply unhappy, for whatever reason, people for whom life is, for a bit, a struggle, then it seems that almost everyone acknowledges suicidal thoughts, if only fleetingly. It's a question I ask almost every working day. 'Do you ever think about harming yourself then? To the extent of making plans? How would you do it then? What would stop you?' and, almost always, people pause before answering, as they consider the level of honesty that this question demands, and then say 'Yes ... but...' The question is intended, obviously, not to *encourage* but to *prevent*. Rather like discussing contraception with a 13-year-old – allowing that door to be opened, being generous, without judgement and with proper compassion. It may feel risky, but it's also much safer. It tends to prevent the thing that we are naming. But it's not a question I used to ask every day of a person who is *actually dying*.

'What is it you're most frightened of then, Jim?'
    'I'm frightened of carrying on like this. I'm frightened of *not* dying.'
    Silence.
    'That's my bottom line, Doctor,' says Jim, anticipating what would be my next question. 'I don't want to be left like this. It's shite.'

This is the problem with Gawande's humane questions. The problem with them is that they make communication *much better*. And if you promise, implicitly, to accompany someone to the edge of their lives, you have an obligation to go where they take you. And the view down, from where I'm standing here with Jim, is vertiginous.

I think that I know and understand the best arguments against a doctor helping someone like Jim with what he *really* seems to want.

Argument #1

He doesn't *really* want it. It's the symptoms talking, not the person. The best version of Jim would be horrified if he knew that he was bothering his doctor with such questions. The doctor's job is to use his skill to help Jim to find that best version of himself again, and listen to *him* instead. So: does Jim have any treatable symptoms? Any treatable factors that are impairing his decision-making? There are many, potentially, and all should to be explored. Pain and distress are the most obvious, though he denies them, and will continue to deny them for the rest of his life, even when, towards the end, he is clearly experiencing both. 'He'll never tell you, Doctor,' as Adie says. Constipation? Urinary retention? Wrong drugs? Calcium levels in blood too high? Sodium too low? Brain metastases? All possible. All, to some extent, treatable.

Jim is bereaved. *So*, asks my inner voice, *have you considered offering Jim counselling for his grief? Would he benefit from anti-depressants?* Jim's life lost all purpose on the day that Margaret died. He doesn't admit to feeling low, and is uninterested in exploring his feelings of grief, however gently and carefully I try to ask. He sees these questions – and all such questions really – as an intrusion, a distraction. I persevere, nonetheless, feeling as I do that I am disrespecting his one clearly stated desire, which was not to be messed around by doctors.

We doctors, I think it is fair to say, are happier with the kinds of complex classification systems that we have invented in order to describe and categorise human suffering, and most of the time this scientific model of classification and study makes for powerful tools to help us in the alleviation of pain. However, we are often less accepting of people's own formulations: in Jim's case – 'I don't want to be left like this. It's shite.' I risk, in interpreting Jim's suffering as *something to be treated*, turning it into something else – something technical; something easier. More tractable, more sciency, but no longer, in essence, Jim's suffering. I could go deeper. I could argue that an attempt to separate an idealised Jim from the reality of his suffering and respect *him* is to raise all sorts of unanswerable Platonic questions about what constitutes that perfect or essential idea of Jim whose will I ought to be respecting. And the answer seems likely to be, that I should be respecting that version of Jim who is content to die in the manner mandated by society, and is less inclined to ask disagreeable questions of me. I'm cherry-picking my ideal Jim – choosing the conformist Jim over the inconvenient, cussed old bugger, who is looking up at me with his watery blue eyes, waiting for an answer. I'm begging the question.

Of course it is absolutely my duty to treat Jim's suffering, provided, of course, that that is what he wants – but I need also to accept that this may result in a Jim even more determined, and more capable, of taking control of the nature, the when, the where and the how, of the end of his life. This may all seem rather theoretical but, sitting opposite the real Jim, who smells of smoke and Brut, who is scared, and who is growing visibly impatient as I question him, it seems like a misappropriation. Jim has no time for my exegesis of his suffering.

Argument #2
There is something about life which is valuable beyond the thoughts, interests and feelings of the person doing the living. This idea, of the inherent value of life – that life is sacred – feels emotionally plausible. To say that life is sacred is to present an argument so apparently strong that it effectively ends the argument. But it raises many questions too. It seems to imply the

existence of some personhood or god whose valuation of a life is more important than the value placed on that life by the person whose life it is.

I find speculating about the place of consciousness in the universe fascinating and fun, but it's irrelevant if I'm trying to answer the question, of why, even if awareness does exist in some form out with our own heads, that could tell us anything useful about the value of Jim's life beyond the value that he puts upon it. If God speaks suddenly, loudly and clearly to Jim, and to me, and tells us that Jim's life *is* valuable, and yet Jim still persists in his view that it isn't, who or what is to arbitrate between Jim's view, and God's?

As it happens, Jim has a minister. I met him, a few weeks later, in Jim's front room. A man in his early forties wearing a fleece with a church logo – a fish, a net, a cross – on the chest. No ecclesiastical collar, no black suit, but a winning, familiar manner about him. He drank tea, and prayed with Jim and Adie, whom he clearly knew well, brought comfort, watched a little telly with them, then left. I asked Jim about it. 'I didn't know that you were a church-goer, Jim?' And he said he was, both he and Margaret had gone to the fisherman's mission, until Margaret died. Then he nodded at Adie, who was in the kitchen, washing the tea cup. 'It's for her really. I'm not bothered, but she likes that kind of stuff.'

Argument #3

Far less fraught than the last, though similar, this argument states that the problem is not with respecting Jim's wishes as such, just supposing we can be sufficiently certain about what Jim's wishes really are, and whether he *really* means what he's saying. The problem lies with the effects that Jim's decision might have on other people. If we lived in a society in which people were permitted to determine the circumstances of the ends of their lives, the consequences of this would make our society intolerable. Reasons for this are many. It would impose an intolerable pressure on the old and the sick to decide the timing of the ending of their lives to suit the timetable and convenience of others. Indeed, given the exponentially rising costs of looking after the dependent elderly in nursing homes, I think that you might reasonably expect a subtle intensification of pressure on elderly dependent people to 'do the decent thing', if that facility were available and de-stigmatised. It would inevitably have the effect of making assisted dying, for example, less extraordinary. You might reasonably expect that if provision were made under stringent safeguards for assisted dying for those whose lives were, say, intolerable and nearing an end, then inevitably there would be pressure for these safeguards to be relaxed. Questions would be raised about what constitutes 'intolerable', and 'near', and then drift to more fundamental questions about why we need these stringent safeguards in the first place. If the only motivation for enabling assisted dying is to respect the settled desire of those people who no longer value continued living, then having conditions such as 'intolerable suffering' and being 'almost dead anyway' are extraneous. What counts are people's settled, authentic wishes.

These are very real concerns. The 'slippery slope' argument, which as an argument is common, and commonly abused, seems plausibly applied here: in those countries where assisted dying has become accepted, the effect has, indeed, been that it has become normalised, and it is argued, in the Netherlands at least, that indications for assisted dying have become progressively less stringent. The issue of vulnerable people being pressurised into accepting assisted dying for reasons of money or convenience doesn't seem to be such a big issue yet, but economic circumstances are changing, and not for the better, at least as far as the vulnerable elderly are concerned.

But this argument depends for its effect on adopting a certain perspective. It starts from an assumption that it is acceptable to deprive people of the remains of their autonomy when it comes to determining the circumstances of the end of their lives. We could just as easily start with the opposite assumption. We could imagine a society where it was absolutely the norm that people were permitted to determine the circumstances of the ending of their own lives, and that this was, indeed, a fundamental kind of right, and that to infringe that right would be considered to be outrageous and wrong. We could then imagine that in that society a responsible movement might grow, advocating the restriction of access to this right to determine the circumstances of the end of your own life, by, say, children, or those under the influence of alcohol or drugs, or the emotionally disturbed, or transiently mentally ill. Rather like the kinds of restrictions we have on people getting a tattoo. People need to be protected against flippant choices. I know I do.

Practically everybody would agree, I think, that these sorts of restrictions would be very wise indeed. But they would also give rise to a second debate within that society about how to determine how far to restrict people's access to assisted dying. Whether depriving certain people in certain circumstances of the right to end their own lives, in fact amounted to a 'slippery slope' towards depriving people of this right altogether. It seems that this form of argument – the 'slippery slope' – in fact assumes its own conclusion. It begs the question.

———

'So I've got eight weeks left. I want to go to that place in Switzerland. What's it called?'

'Dignitas?'

'That's the one. I've got £1000 in the bank. Will that be enough?'

'I … don't know…'

Jim looks at me as if I'm stupid. He looks at the computer on my desk, and then at the mobile phone beside it.

'Can you not just check?'

'Ah … sure.' I bring up Google. I type 'Dignitas Zurich' in the search box. I stop before clicking.

'I'm not sure if I'm allowed to do this.'

'Allowed? I thought that you were a doctor.'

'I … am…' I say, beginning to doubt the fact myself. We sit a moment in uneasy silence, Jim looking disappointed now, as well as frightened. His doctor, me, having promised so much, seems to be bailing at the first sign of trouble.

'Do *you* not have a …'

'*Computer?* Nah. I leave all that stuff to Adie. But I can't ask her about *this*. She'll just say no. Or stall, until it's too late.'

Uneasy silence, which I find intolerable. But it's intolerable not to help him, either.

'Have you thought about asking at the public library?' I say, knowing as I make this suggestion how small it makes me.

I call a helpline.

Doctors facing legal difficulties have access to a defence organisation, for which we pay several thousand pounds a year. I speak to a sympathetic woman who listens intently to my story, and understands my predicament.

'So what can I do, within the law, to help Jim in the way he wants to be helped?'

She is kind, and realistic. The answer is, 'absolutely nothing'.

I have already gone too far; I have already crossed a line, by suggesting that a public librarian might help Jim to Google 'Dignitas'. She thinks that I probably needn't worry, but if I had done the Googling myself, then I would certainly be potentially guilty of a criminal offence, of aiding and abetting a suicide. She told me that I shouldn't help Jim in any way. I shouldn't give any information to Dignitas, even with Jim's consent, and that includes giving Jim copies of his medical records, even though he is entitled to them, for any other reason. If Jim asks for my signature on his passport application, then I need to contact them again, for more legal advice. All these things are a part of a slippery slope towards Physician Assisted Suicide, which is illegal. And I shouldn't Google 'Dignitas' when I get home, either. If everything goes wrong and I find myself in court, my online search history becomes evidence.

I ask to speak with her boss. He is much less nice, and agrees with everything that the last person has told me.

I say words to the effect that 'this seems wholly wrong to me. It's my duty to help Jim in every way I can, and most especially now that he's dying, and relying on me ... If I do what I think is right, go against your advice, and help him anyway, what will happen?'

These things always come out in the end, one way or another, or so he tells me. I'll be guilty of a criminal offence. I'll lose my licence to practise, and probably get a suspended gaol sentence, if I'm lucky. And they won't pay for my criminal defence barrister, either.

Argument #4

So it seems that there's a fourth argument, much less celebrated than the others, unrecognised really, and not really much of an argument at all.

It's about being too scared to do what you know is right. About not doing something because it is overwhelmingly inconvenient. It's about failing in your duty because you are intimidated by a law which seems to you to be bent and cramped, distorted and incoherent, and shouldn't apply to you at all, but does.

Two weeks later, Jim went to the library, got an address, wrote a letter to Dignitas, and sent it. The phone number he'd been given on the computer was out of date – or he thinks he might have written one of the numbers down wrongly. Before he got a reply though, and a few weeks after having written, I was called to his house by Adie. He had become quite suddenly, extremely agitated. He had coughed up a lot of blood that morning, and his breathlessness had become abruptly worse. He was pacing up and down his sitting room, unable to sit for more than an instant. He seemed to be in pain. He had hit her when she tried to calm him, not hard, more of a fly swat, but all the same. He was frightened of dying. Couldn't stand living – pacing the room, saying, 'This is shite, I can't take another two weeks of *this…*' He was frightened of being admitted to hospital, or a hospice. He was frightened of bleeding to death, or asphyxiating, which is a common and reasonable fear for those who are dying of lung cancer. He was frightened of doctors, frightened of me, and what I might do to him. He was frightened of dying, and frightened of being alive.

He had no obvious, reversible causes for his agitation, other than fear and suffocation. I gave him an injection – some morphine for his breathlessness, and some tranquiliser for his fear, and laid in a large store of injectables for the rocky days ahead. But with the help of his daughter, and her inexhaustible love, and a small team of nurses, we got him through the last, worse days. We gave him large doses of opiates as he grew more breathless, and more tranquilisers. He wasn't agitated, didn't experience any more of that awful fear, but he wasn't the same person either. He died, quietly, bang on schedule, two weeks later. It wasn't a bad death, really, and he died at home. But it wasn't the death that Jim had wanted.

The Problem of Alicia's Smile

When Alicia was tiny, her mother maintains she was normal in her development, but I have my doubts. They have pictures of her as a two-year-old, sitting propped up on her father's lap, looking up into the camera, smiling. Or perhaps it was simply a grimace, a reflex from that tiny shock of the light of the sun touching her face. The smile she wears in these photos is not so different from the one she has now, 15 years later: whenever a new person comes into her room; when her long hair is brushed until it shines or the soft toys which surround her are rearranged; when she is dressed in her favourite primrose yellow pyjamas – or even when she is subjected to blood tests, or has her catheter changed. But when she smiles, her mother and her carers smile back and make a fuss of her: they say that Alicia likes it when her sheets are straightened, or the curtain is drawn back to welcome the new day. It seems that Alicia welcomes her mother, or her brother, or the doctor, or the lady that cleans her room, because she smiles whenever anyone comes in. They say that Alicia is brave: and it's true, that every day she greets every new indignity with the same smile.

Alicia had problems, it seems, pretty much from birth. I didn't know her then, but I know her well now, and on a number of occasions I have had to excavate deeply into her medical records and, without particularly intending to, have built up a strong impression of the events of those years. The pregnancy and birth were uncomplicated, but she had been slow to feed. She didn't seem to latch on or swallow well. Her mother, a determined, embattled woman, had wanted to breastfeed, but eventually, with the encouragement of a worried health visitor, had switched to artificial feeds. Alicia's mum felt guilty. The process of giving birth, of breastfeeding, of nurturing her baby was important to her, and she blamed the neonatal medical team for undermining her.

Alicia gained weight, but slowly. Her swallowing troubles worsened, she vomited constantly, and seemed to be inhaling her feeds. She had a significant episode of pneumonia when she was six months old. Just after her second birthday, her mother expressed concern that she wasn't supporting her own weight. Alicia babbled, but she seemed to lack words. Her mother started to interpret for her, turning her vocalisations, which seemed to lack structure or intention, into words and sentences, then whole emotional narratives.

Alicia had always smiled; she had always had a cheery nature. She smiled at everything. Alicia's most resilient characteristic was always this – this *brightness* in her soul.

When she was 30 months old, she started having fits. It had seemed to take days to get her convulsions properly under control. According to her mother, it was then that her developmental problems had begun. I know, in fact, that this isn't the case. Her medical records clearly indicate that her parents had been concerned by her lack of developmental 'milestones' well before her first major episode. Indeed there is evidence of concern that she had been having minor convulsions for months before her first admission, but something about Alicia's mother makes it impossible to challenge. It would seem as if I were being heartless, or, in some way, disloyal.

Her father, a university professor, left the parental home when Alicia was eight, and is now a distant, if caring, presence. Her mother is highly protective of a certain chronological view of her daughter's problems. 'Until *this* happened, Alicia could do…' whatever … but now she can't.

It is a narrative unflattering towards the medical profession, who have always been one step behind Alicia and her problems – late in diagnosis, late in reacting to change, insistent on immunisations, medications and treatments that have only brought complications, side effects and harm, and always slow to accept responsibility or blame. Alicia's mother has interposed herself between Alicia and a dangerous and indifferent world. Alicia's mother can be suspicious, highly protective, even hostile. Around her, you tread gently.

Every month I take blood from Alicia. This is part of a negotiation, between the hospital, her parents, and me. Alicia is fed via a jejunostomy tube, a tube fed through her abdominal wall directly into her gut. She is fed overnight, and has been for many years, because she no longer swallows reliably at all. She is susceptible to deficiencies in vitamins and micro-nutrients which have to be watched for diligently. Her convulsions are suppressed by a cocktail of anti-convulsants which tend to conflict with her other medications and these conflicts are exacerbated by her diminished kidney function, so blood levels of these have to be regularly monitored. There is suspicion that Alicia's mother feeds her vitamin and mineral supplements of unknown provenance via her jejunostomy, at night, when no one can see, and that these unknown factors might destabilise

Alicia's drug and metabolic balance further. I have become something of an expert in getting blood from Alicia, although it's a job I dread.

She sits up in bed. Her curtains are open spilling light into the room. Her long, flaxen hair is spread out on the pillow around her. There is a poster of the cast from *Friends* on the wall facing her. Ross is deemed her favourite. There is another separate poster of Ross, with his glossy black hair and his vulnerable puppy smile. Her mother, always there for her, is tying a pale blue ribbon in her hair. Every morning Alicia's mother fixes her daughter's hair. In recent years she has tried a little make-up, and today there is a hint of lilac eyeshadow, which I notice is the same as her mother's.

Alicia's skin is thin and almost translucent. She has tiny, spidery veins which seem to float just under the skin. I say, 'Hello, Alicia, how are you?' and Alicia smiles and vocalises. In the crook of her left elbow is her current favourite soft toy, a little dog. Her mother answers on her daughter's behalf. 'Hello, Doctor, we're fine!' And I remove from my bag the fine butterfly needle, blood bottles and tourniquet, and Alicia gazes up at the ceiling, which she always does, whatever else is happening, whoever else is in the room.

'What's it today then, Doctor?' asks Alicia's mother, smiling brightly, and I say, 'Usual! Kidney, liver, drug levels, blood counts...' and her mother, as she has for years, writes down my answers in a spiral bound book, 'Alicia's Medical Diary', which she keeps always ready on a cabinet by her bed.

Her mother clasps Alicia's other hand tightly, whispers urgently and reassuringly into her daughter's ear, and winces when I slip the needle in, as if it is her skin that I am piercing and not her daughter's. Alicia smiles at the roof. Most times I get the blood sample without too much problem, but sometimes not. Sometimes a bloom of blood spreads around the vein which I have just burst, and I withdraw the needle and press firmly. Nowadays I never try more than once. In the past I would become increasingly agitated as I tried a second or third time with diminishing hope of success, my mood in tune with Alicia's mother's, who would mutter wordlessly, her hands growing white and bloodless as she squeezed her daughter's.

'Well done, Alicia!' I chirp, whether I have succeeded or failed, pressing cotton wool to the wound. 'You're brave!' Alicia's eyes are half closed; she is dozing now, gone from the world, although the smile remains, flickering on and off.

'Thank you, Doctor,' says her mother, gazing into her daughter's face, moving a lock of Alicia's hair from her forehead.

My heart is like a stone in my chest after I have seen Alicia. I always feel angry. I don't really know who I am treating, or why. I don't think that it can be Alicia, because I don't think that Alicia knows, or cares, one way or another. During the long years when her paediatricians tried to make a precise diagnosis for Alicia, brain imaging certainly seemed to suggest abnormalities so profound that they cast doubt on Alicia's capacity to have any higher brain function at all. I don't know for sure whether she feels pain, or distress – I have never seen evidence of it – but her mother certainly maintains that she does, and it's safer, surely, to proceed on the assumption that her mother is right; but simply avoiding pain and distress doesn't justify a fraction of the medical interventions that have been performed to keep Alicia as she is.

I think, in fact, that I'm probably treating her mother. Or perhaps the team of carers who help her mother, who collude, brilliantly, compassionately, wholeheartedly, in the theatre of personhood that is performed around their patient. Perhaps I am simply doing what I'm told by her hospital consultants and a medical system that is invested in maintaining Alicia as she is. But every time anyone perpetrates even the tiniest discomfort upon Alicia, it is done to benefit someone else, and I wonder, has anyone even thought about that? And whose job would it be anyway to think about it?

The truth is I don't even know whether there is a person in there to treat.

———

On a good day, I am successful and have three blood bottles to send off. My visit to Alicia has taken 15 minutes or so and I get back to my office quickly. I always have more stuff to do. Still a little angry with the world, I sign a death certificate, mandating the burning of the body of a man I knew slightly, who died, peacefully, at home. I take the greatest care over this, even though my patient is dead. Caring about dead people is important. I don't really know why, but it is. If you mess up a death certificate, it delays funerals, can demolish crematoria, leads to unnecessary autopsies and angry conversations with coroners and fiscals. It causes enormous pain to so many. Mangled death certificates have caused me sleepless nights, and today I am angry and out of sorts, and prone to error.

I speak with the daughter of an elderly woman with dementia in a nursing home whom I am treating for pneumonia. Mrs Sturgess is likely to die tonight. Both her daughter, Rita, and I have agreed to 'keep her comfortable' this time, but I still want to check in with her, make sure that Rita is still happy with this: no more admissions, no more antibiotics, no more unnecessary distress. She is happy. I am happy. It feels right. Although I am very fond of Mrs Sturgess, who had been a dancer in her youth, and had a photo of herself, a glam 75 in spangles and lycra, on her mantel shelf in the nursing home, now, at the end of her life, it feels like we are all doing the right thing.

I have tea with Nadja, my trainee. She is unhappy. I always look forward to having tea with Nadja, who is clever and reflective, cares a lot about things that matter, and is just a little lazy about dealing with things that don't. She is unhappy because she has had a request from a 19-year-old, Charmaine, requesting a termination of pregnancy. This is the kind of thing that matters very much indeed. Nadja has no doubt that she can legally grant this: the law in the UK, deliberately or otherwise, is structured in such a way that, providing the request is made reasonably early on in the pregnancy, the termination can always be medically justified. Nadja has beliefs about the world, largely inherited, but important to her nonetheless, that forbid abortion. Nonetheless, she has no doubt that she *will* grant it. Charmaine herself has no doubt that this is what she wants, and it is her body, after all. But Charmaine had seemed quite flippant in her request. She has a child already: Robbie, a three-year-old, who, during this most delicate conversation, ran wild, screaming at his mother or ransacking cupboards and drawers until placated by Nadja's smartphone, which was sticky now with toddler goo. And Charmaine had had a previous termination of pregnancy after Robbie's birth, and had been started on the pill, but hadn't taken it because it had made her moody and she was worried about becoming fat.

Nadja is unhappy because she had felt herself becoming angry with her patient. Charmaine had chewed on gum throughout the consultation; she had seemed indifferent, even cold towards her wild son who had tried to cling to Nadja after they had left.

Nadja hadn't shown any of this anger. Charmaine was poor and undereducated, and Nadja is neither. Nadja is too good a doctor to give her patient a hard time because she's pissed off with her. She is unhappy because she can't figure out *why* she's so angry; what her anger is telling her.

'If it's okay to do the abortion once, then it's okay to do it twice,' she says. 'I mean there are obviously better ways of managing her. Her care isn't exactly a triumph of medicine, but that's not *her* fault. And if it's not okay to do the abortion, then we shouldn't have done it the first time round. The gum chewing is irrelevant. I just don't understand ... I shouldn't feel so riled about it.'

Nadja is often tired in the mornings. She has an 18-month-old at home, and she and her partner work part-time to ensure that there is always somebody to pick up Sammy in the evening. Nadja's days are pressured at both ends in ways that mine no longer are. But no matter how little she has slept, Nadja always pitches up to work in the mornings.

Hungry. Angry. Late. Tired. This is the mantra we repeat to one another – know this about yourself and you avoid your worst mistakes in medicine, and today it seems we are both angry.

I find myself offloading in turn to Nadja. Teatime at my work is often like this. Questions of life and death, in the slow lane.

'What is it,' I say, 'that bugs me so, about looking after Alicia? What is it about her smile that so disturbs?'

'Why is it,' asks Nadja, 'that some bodies seem to matter, and others don't?'

And how are we to tell the difference?

———

I once tried to have this conversation, or something like it, with Alicia's mother.

Alicia had had a series of short admissions over the previous few months, for what seemed on the face of it to be minor problems – more, and more prolonged convulsions, or vomiting, or new transient grimaces, different from her usual smile, which her mother interpreted as distress. Whenever she went into hospital, she would be assaulted with needles and tubes, multiple blood tests, scans, x-rays, endoscopies, and would come home paler, more listless, no better. The hospital was suspicious of Alicia's mother, or at least she perceived it to be. Many years previously, Alicia's mother had threatened to take Alicia home from hospital before she was recovered from a bout of pneumonia, and her then consultant, fearful that the child would die, had threatened to involve social services to compel Alicia to stay. The damage to the relationship had never been repaired. Now, whenever illness threatened, her mother would weep bitter tears, cling to her daughter like an animal to its cub. While the ambulance was called, the nursing staff in the most gentle way would have to detach her mother from her daughter, limb by limb, finger by finger, so that the ambulance technicians could transfer her. At least this is how the nurses described it. They struggled with Alicia's mother. Everyone dreaded Alicia's illnesses. The very air around Alicia seemed to crackle with hostility and love.

I say, 'Alicia's health is very vulnerable.'

We are three: myself, and opposite me, Alicia's mother, holding her daughter's hand. Between us, Alicia, looking up at the roof, smiling.

'I know.'

It occurs to me that I have known these two for almost 10 years. Yet mother and daughter are as opaque to me as on the morning I met them.

'Sometimes when she gets really unwell, it can be difficult to know what to do.'

She says nothing. I think she trusts me, which is why I have been mandated to have this conversation.

'... that's why, sometimes, when she's really ill, she *has* to go to hospital. I'd like to talk about what we should do the next time Alicia needs to go to hospital.'

'Alicia doesn't like hospital.'

This time I say nothing.

She says again, 'Alicia *hates* hospitals.' I nod, non-committally, thinking: *you. You hate hospitals.*

'I know what you're thinking, Doctor.'

It always irritates me when people say this. When people say this, they're always wrong.

'*You* don't think there's anyone in there. You think there's no one home.' She turns to Alicia, a smile on her face. 'The doctor thinks we don't understand a thing that he says, but *I* know we do.'

But she's not wrong in this case. That is *exactly* what I'm thinking. I think that Alicia perceives some things, and nothing more. Light, hunger, pain, touch, love, perhaps. But I would never say that, to anyone. Too cruel. So I find yet again that I have nothing to say.

'Only *I* know when she's sick, and only *I* know when she's well.'

She taps the side of her head with her forefinger, the old fashioned 'nutcase' gesture. 'Power of love, Doctor. It's the power of love.' Like I'd know nothing about that.

Is Alicia only valuable because she is *loved?* Do babies just matter because we love them? And if they are unloved, do they no longer matter?

If Alicia weren't loved, like Charmaine's foetus, say, would that make her morally indifferent?

When Rita and I agreed that Mrs Sturgess had reached the end of her life, and that there was no merit in prescribing treatment to prolong her dying, did we do that because we cared about her any less?

———

Nadja filled out the necessary forms to arrange for Charmaine's termination of pregnancy, but Charmaine never picked them up. A couple of weeks later, she saw Nadja again. She had changed her mind. What she hadn't managed to say to Nadja the first time, was that she had just split with her boyfriend, her three-year-old's father. She was fed up, stressed out and couldn't cope. Robbie, the child, was driving her nuts, and she couldn't bear to think of having another. But now she was back together with her man and her perspective was changed. She couldn't quite believe what she had been planning to do – she was crying, according to Nadja, tears of relief as she said this. 'It's like I was planning to kill my own baby!' And she certainly wasn't chewing gum anymore. She said thank you to Nadja for talking her out of the abortion, though Nadja had no memory at all of trying to do so. The three-year-old was being looked after by his dad, who was playing with him rather noisily outside in the waiting room, but no one much minded. Charmaine seemed happier, warmer in her manner, cooperative and engaged, and already wearing a glazed and far-off expression on her face, her right hand drifting towards her tummy as she talked about the baby that she was going to keep.

———

Alicia died suddenly just after her 16th birthday. From time to time, her vomiting would increase, she would become dehydrated and need hospital admission for re-hydration. It was thought that she was having intermittent episodes of bowel obstruction due to a twisting of her small intestine – small bowel volvulus. She never had sufficient resilience for this to be definitively treated, and, besides, years and years of medical complexity had left her mother averse to having her daughter messed around by doctors. She had developed bile-stained vomiting, eventually been admitted to hospital, where she had been assessed by the medical team, and sent home, because she had seemed to be settling. Alicia, according to her mother, was always distressed by hospitals, and always wanted to be home as soon as possible. But she had collapsed later that night at home, becoming feverish, dry, vomiting uncontrollably, and seeming less alert. By the time she was readmitted, she was very sick. She had irreversible damage to most of her small intestine, was developing septic shock which wasn't responding to antibiotics, and was clearly dying. Her mother, bereft, had sat with her through the night, holding her hand, fixing her hair, watching as her daughter slipped away.

It was obvious in hindsight that Alicia should never have been sent home. At the time of discharge, she already had had a flicker of fever, her pulse and breathing were up, she just wasn't 'right'. But the consultant looking after her seemed not to have taken proper account of this, or if she had, hadn't been clear or explicit enough in her reasons for deciding to let Alicia go. An internal hospital enquiry affirmed culpability: it was one of these medical disasters which doctors dread, that happen so easily, that so blight our lives. Blame was apportioned to many doctors and nurses, some of whom went off work sick with the misery and remorse from having let their patient down.

Alicia's mother was more forgiving than the hospital administration. She said afterwards that, although it was important that people learn from their mistakes, they shouldn't be punished. What mattered was that her daughter had had a good life while she lived – a wonderful life. She had been surrounded by people who loved her and cared for her. Her death was just a tiny sad part of something that was much bigger, and ultimately beautiful. We all have something to learn from the way Alicia approached her life, at least that's what her mother thought. So she wasn't going to give in to anger or bitterness or blame. She would wipe away her tears, and she would carry on. And she could tell, from the smile that her daughter had worn right up to the moment of her death, that that was what Alicia would have wanted.

How to be Good

Theo didn't seem to realise that it was *me* he was talking to.

Perhaps it was because he had been kept waiting on the line, but all that I could hear in his voice was impatience. He had told my receptionist that it was an emergency – although it clearly wasn't – but I had been with a patient, so he had had to wait. He didn't recognise my voice, although I recognised his, almost immediately. He had an Ulster accent – a gentle, cultured, persuasive voice. He had been my student for a few months, a few years ago. He had shown extraordinary promise. He was only twenty something then, but he had a kind of authority about him, a gentleness, a commanding, caring, grown-up manner that made him unusually appealing to the patients he saw. He was knowledgeable, humble, keen and able to learn. I remembered him well because of the kinds of conversations that we had had – a passionate, engaged difference about almost everything that mattered – and his respect for me, mine for him, despite the difference in age and status. I remembered him because he was the best student that I ever had.

'Hi, this is Theo Irving, Medical Registrar, St Mary's, I need to speak with the duty doc?'

'That's me.'

The same gentle voice, but there's an edge to it today. He's in a rush. This being, doubtless, one of a million transactions he's got to cope with this evening. Clearly it's not the time for *Hi Theo! You remember me? The one that gave you 82 per cent in your clinical exam and a full bonus 10 marks for compassion and caring?* It wasn't that kind of day.

'What's the emergency?'

'I don't know if you know her. It's about a Mrs Caitlen Dalrymple, date of birth November 12th 1928?'

I open her notes on my desktop. Of course I know her. Memorable name. An energetic 88-year-old with a hobbling gait and a stick. She had a hip replacement a few years ago, and for a few weeks I visited her regularly at home. She had a touch of heart failure that complicated her care, making her ankles swell like water sacks – dropsy, as it once was called. Legs sloshing around in their skins, she hobbled from room to room in her bungalow, waving her stick expansively at the garden window as she gave us a virtual tour of her brightly coloured peonies. I have a feeling that this might even have been during the time of Theo's attachment with us. I think that he might have known her too. She recovered remarkably quickly from her hip. She was on anticoagulants to slow her blood clotting. Her heart failure had caused an irregular pulse, which put her at risk of blood clots and consequent stroke. She needed bloods done from time to time to check that we had the dose of her warfarin right. An undemanding lady. Sometimes, if the weather was good, she would be in her wellies in the garden, flourishing under the warmer weather, as old people do, and I would kneel down among the roses with her to take her blood, enjoy a bit of sun, a bit of outdoors. These are little moments that punctuate a day, brighten it, if you can make the time to notice them.

'I do know her. What's the emergency?'

'She's coming home tonight. She's had a really rocky time in hospital. Her clotting's been all over the place and she's had a couple of major bleeds from stress ulcers. I don't know if you know, but she's been diagnosed with a gall bladder cancer? It's not treatable so she's for palliative care, but she's not too symptomatic yet. The main thing is her clotting. It's been really hard to stabilise so she probably needs daily bloods to get it right.'

I know he's pressured, and this is one job of many, but his speech is rushed and his voice is a little raised. He's not quite rude, but he's not really leaving any gaps for me to say anything, and that little questioning up-flick at the end of each sentence, where he's suggesting I might see my way to visiting this vulnerable elderly lady at the end of her life who can't cope alone, just to get her bloods right. It makes him sound anxious, a little out of control, passive-aggressive even. He's spreading his stress around. A bad quality in a doctor. It's exactly the kind of trait I like to discuss with students. It's a good thing to know about yourself if you're doing it. It's a good thing to stop doing. I'm maybe setting the bar a bit high here, but that *was* Theo's bar. This isn't quite the Theo I used to know.

'It doesn't sound much like an emergency to me. Sounds like she needs just to stay in hospital a day or two longer to get her bloods right.'

This is in fact a little mischievous of me. There is an un-spoken rule governing this kind of interaction between medical colleagues. The context of this conversation, the overarching set of assumptions and rules that govern our behaviour – the *paradigm* – is that there are always too few resources and too many patients. Too many people, too many needs that can't be met. No one is prepared to raise the taxes or borrow the money that would be necessary to alleviate the problem, and even if they did, that might prove to be unsustainable as a solution. Everyone's getting older after all, developing more and more complex illness, and the taxable population isn't growing fast enough to keep up. So there are too few beds in hospitals, too few nurses and those that there are labour under a punitively hierarchical system that destroys their capacity for care. For those that make it out alive, social care provision is terrible, and people pile up in hospital beds just because there isn't the money to pay for people to care for them at home. If you have cancer, say, or renal failure, or you are a child, or you are multiply injured in a car pile-up, or aren't too ill and have a great GP, you might be okay. If you are elderly and are chronically ill with multiple, complex, interacting pathologies, or if you have any kind of psychiatric problem or substance issue, then provision is so thin and inflexible that it might be better if we were to liberate ourselves from all illusion and stop pretending that we *had* a system. I'm over-stating the case. Perhaps.

The unspoken rule is this: while it's okay to moan about all this in private with understanding colleagues, it's not okay to hold them to account for bad medical decisions and shoddy behaviours, which are forced on them by a broken system and an ungenerous electorate. So when I imply to Theo that he might keep Mrs Dalrymple in hospital longer in order to fix her properly, I'm being unfair. They need the beds to warehouse other patients. Theo just doesn't have the power to keep her in. And because we exist within the transparent walls of this set of assumptions – we doctors, we patients, the all-inclusive we – we stop seeing them. We stop seeing them as walls. They become normal to us. We accept them for what they are – that set of rules governing our available behaviours.

There's a little silence on the line. The above, unstated of course, but lying there like a corpse between us all the same.

'She needs to get home. She's been in hospital for six weeks.'

This is a good point. A good-*ish* point. A standard move in this particular game. Hospitals are lethal environments for the old. Every day that goes by for an older person in hospital is a day lost – another day of passivity, immobility, gathering despair, of institutionalisation, incontinence, the risk of falls, lethal infection, diarrhoea, boredom, drug error, unnecessary medical investigation and loss of freedom. A step closer to chronic dependency, or death, or death-in-life. We admit people to hospital all the time for the shakiest reasons, with minimal thought, as if it were the neutral, somehow harmless, option. When we admit a potentially dependent person to hospital, or decide to keep them there, it should be with the gravity of a good young surgeon opening an abdomen: it is so commonly the terminal decision in a person's life. I think I might already, in the distant past, have shared all this with Theo.

I have on my desktop Mrs Dalrymple's opened medical records, in electronic form, of course. The reason that she is on anticoagulants is because her irregular heartbeat puts her at a higher risk of a future stroke, and anticoagulants reduce this risk, but at the price of an indeterminate risk of bleeding – possibly bleeding to death, if she has a fall or cracks her head. This is such a common medical scenario, this dilemma, to treat, or not to treat, that my computer desktop comes equipped with a little calculator in the corner, telling me what her annual risk of having a stroke is. Mrs Dalrymple's risk is

5 per cent. That's 0.01 per cent per day. Too high, if it were me. But Mrs D already has an 80-plus per cent risk of dying this year anyway, whatever we do. So what risk would be too high for *her*?

'Why don't you just stop the anticoagulants?' I suggest.

'She was reviewed on the ward round this morning. It's all been discussed. Her consultant physician was quite clear that she needed to stay on the warfarin.' Theo's sounding testy now. When someone's argument is based on an appeal to authority, they have no argument. Having no strong argument of your own is a common source of discomfort among young doctors.

'But!' I say, 'Her annual stroke risk is 5 per cent, her life expectancy is...' but I stop myself, buffeted as I am by the high-volume thought waves coming down the telephone: *Just fecking do it! Lazy fecking bar-steward! Just fecking...* Although, on reflection, Theo would never use, or even think to use these kinds of words.

It must have been four or five years ago when he had been my student.

The reason that I admired Theo, or part of it anyway, was for his capacity to think a problem through from the bottom up, without reaching for too many assumptions, too many off-the-peg points of view or solutions. Another was that he was fun to talk to. I like to talk with people about ideas, but I'm not always terribly good at telling when others share my interest. Theo did *seem* to share my interest.

We are driving to a patient's house for an emergency visit one evening, a late house call. It is winter and dark and we are driving into one of the grimmer, rain-hammered sink estates that surround my place of work.

When the call came in, a few hours earlier, I had already been feeling jaded and annoyed. I often was at that stage in the afternoon. As I drift toward the end of a busy day, I become less open to the possibility of events that might disrupt the possibility of getting home. It isn't just me that is affected like this. I don't think I'm unusually bad in this respect. It's a potent source of error in medical practice, which all doctors and nurses are aware of, or should be. Errors happen at the beginnings and especially the ends of shifts.

There was a voice yelling down the phone at me. A frightened man, I could tell, dressing his fear up as rage.

'It's Debbie. She cannae move her leg. She's had a stroke or something. She's just lying there, screaming and shouting that she cannae move her leg. Are you coming?'

Debbie's husband, or partner, or uncle, or boyfriend, is in his mid-thirties and quite a few years older than she is. He's aggressive, and sounds a bit pissed. He's an alcoholic and on a prescription for opiates and gabapentin, a kind of not-very-effective-but-formidably-spacy painkiller which fetches quite a price in the blocks where he lives. I'm absolutely sure that he's been selling them on, but have never addressed the issue. This is a common situation: a common deception and one that hammers the doctor with feelings of pointlessness and futility. Being in such a prescribing relationship with a patient undermines your integrity like little else. It's not that I've given up, or don't care: quite the contrary. It's that I have so many patients who have been badly prescribed, and it takes so long to undo prescribing harm once it has started that I have a long queue, and I tend to try to manage the easier ones first. Debbie's boyfriend's aggression works as a really powerful disincentive to care.

'Are you coming or not?'

I could hear her shouting in the background: 'When's he fucking coming! Ah cannae move ma leg!'

I am quite resistant at the best of times to visiting people in their houses, especially sweary ones. It's time consuming, and inefficient. Most of the time it's unnecessary. It's always dark inside, if not out; there are always big snuffly dogs; you don't have all the medical records and you never have the right stuff, so it's much more unsafe for the patient. It creates a kind of dependence too – if a person can make it over their threshold, it's almost always better to come to me. If the patient is drunk and aggressive, in my experience, the visit is *almost* always futile. But not always – and that's the problem.

'Sounds like she needs to be looked at. Bring her up to the surgery, I'll see her straight away. She won't even have to wait.'

'You're having a laugh doctor. I'm telling you, she can't walk, and she's in *agony*. She can't even get to the toilet. She's peeing in a bucket! I think she's had a stroke. Or a thrombosis.'

'Well,' I said, suppressing my waves of irritation, 'if you think she's had a stroke, perhaps she needs to be seen in hospital?'

I feel bad about this last bit. A few years ago, the model for how we manage strokes changed from an essentially passive one to one of active management. Because a minority of strokes can be managed by technical medicine, using 'clot-busting' drugs to resupply the affected part of the brain with blood, sometimes with miraculous results, health workers, and the public generally, are encouraged to see stroke as 'Brain Attack!' and send potential patients to hospital as soon as possible for assessment for this treatment. This rebranding is clearly a great thing if you're having stroke. But it has the undesired side effect that when someone in the chain thinks of the word 'stroke', complex, indeterminate, muddled questions become simplified and re-formulated as 'has she had a stroke or not?' The solution then becomes magically apparent. You send her to hospital to have that question answered. The effect is to open a sluice gate for complex social problems to be sent to emergency rooms to have the wrong question answered. It's an example of a dynamic that exists in many other contexts – you see the same with chest pains, vague cancer suspicions, suicidal thoughts or children who might have meningitis. It's one of the reasons that health provision is creaking: too many people sent for specialist care to have the wrong question answered. But I know in my heart that Debbie isn't having a stroke. I would put my house on it. For a start, strokes aren't painful.

'When's he coming? Tell him to get a fucking move on!' called the chorus from the couch.

'We already called an ambulance. They told us to call you.'

I didn't say 'That's a lie'. I didn't say 'It doesn't work like that. If the ambulance crew had really said that, they'd have called me themselves.' Calling adults on lies never works. The most you can do is try to figure out why they're having to lie.

'I'll be an hour or two. Maybe more.'

Rain and sleet lashes the windscreen. It's dark by the time I've finished all my other stuff; late by the time Debbie has surfaced again in my pile of priorities. I sit forward in the car seat trying to clear the glass on the inside. It gets steamed up whenever *I* do. I can't see the house numbers, which seem to have been

perversely jumbled. Debbie and her boyfriend/husband/
uncle/carer live at 105b, and the numbers stop at 104. Every
few yards I stop the car and get out to check. I'd be better off
just sitting down by the gutter sobbing. Theo's presence in the
passenger seat forces me to keep my dignity. I feel I have to set
some kind of example, and sobbing is definitely out. Swearing
too mainly, at least over sustained periods. 105b is on the wrong
side of the road, entrance hidden above a chippie. We've passed
it three times already.

'So Theo, I generally pause for a moment at this point. Collect
my thoughts, reflect on why I'm here, and think a little bit about
what I might encounter, and what we might do, and how we
might do it well.'

We sit for a moment in silence.

In fact, I practically never do this. Sometimes I like to think
that I might – that I might be the kind of person that pauses for
a moment before a hard encounter or a challenge, that I might
be mindful and meditative and focus on my breathing and reflect
for a moment on *why I'm there,* murmuring to myself something
that in another age might have been called prayer but isn't now –
but I never do, and I don't know anyone that does.

I don't know anyone that does – apart from Theo. He comes
closest. Theo is slow and measured in everything he does. He
always seemed to have longer on the ball than the other players.
It's not all words with Theo.

Theo is at the heart of a tiny church – a free, open gathering of
many kinds that meets once a week in his flat or the house of one
of the other members, where they sing and pray and clap and
plan how they might in the week coming do the Lord's work.
He didn't volunteer this to me; I prised it from him during a
different conversation about what we liked to read, or the
music we liked to listen to, or something like that. His house

church sits in a federation of others, each within other churches of different kinds and names, and they coordinate what they do, which is muscular. If they were political, which I suppose they are, Theo's church network would be a militant entryist group, like Christian Trotskyites. It's not just Christians either, of course. They have fraternal groups in the local mosques and Sikh temples too, offering free soup kitchens, crèches, guerrilla gardens in streets and parties for festivals where there is music and face painting, and reaching out to refugees who appear to have nothing, serving folk, irrespective of what they need or deserve or believe or where they come from and what they had to do to get here.

Theo looks at me. I can see, in the hazy yellow light of the street lamp that he is smiling about something. He hesitates and says, 'Yeah. Or we could just get this over with. It's not getting any warmer in your car.'

So we wrap tight against the cold outside, and brave the slippery pee-sprinkled stairwells to the block where Debbie lives.

Theo sees himself, or at least he says he does, as a passive agent in this process of doing his best: he is an empty vessel through which God works his love. All he has to do is be open to that, and the rest will happen. Provided he stays open to the possibility of God working through him, the question of *keeping it up for the long haul* doesn't arise. It is a question of keeping faith, and faith for him is a living thing, an inexhaustible source of joy.

I find this wholly unpersuasive. I am a curmudgeon when it comes to God. Even if there were such a thing, which is an unanswerable question and so, I think, not worth asking, then how would one know whether her promptings were motivated by love, or hate? For those in the world motivated by the promptings of their god, it seems that the latter kind does, often, seem to win out.

'But,' Theo says, 'it's not a question of putting your brains on ice, it's about opening your mind to Him, so that you're prompted to care enough to think about these things in the first place!'

'But,' I say, 'that just displaces the question one step back! If in the end it's your brains that tell you what to do, then whatever your god prompts is irrelevant to the question. What she says doesn't go!'

What's interesting to me is not so much the theology, but the psychology. Why it is that a person as bright, talented and sensitive, and, in all other ways, a person as generally skilled as Theo needs recourse to this illusion or dream, and to supporting arguments which seem so flimsy and self-serving? People like Theo are fascinating to me. I once put the question to him over tea one morning, using much the same words. He smiled, laughed in a non-patronising kind of way, and asked me whether I loved my children, or my wife, or my parents, or indeed anyone much, and then whether I spent a lot of time worrying about whether my relationship with *them* existed, or whether such a question even mattered? And whether their existence in my life was a factor in the sorts of day-to-day decisions I might make about how best to live? And then he said in a kind kind of way that my questioning of his faith was as irrelevant to him as these kinds of questions might be to me. It was a characteristically gentle takedown. I still find Theo's account unpersuasive, but he did seem to get a whole lot more done in life than me.

'Empathy and care have to do with imagination,' I say, my voice ringing out worryingly loud in the empty concrete stair. I am continuing a long conversation that he and I have been having on and off for weeks. How to be good. And why. How to keep it up when no one much wants you to. That is the kind of teaching relationship that we have. The kind of conversation we return to.

Somewhere up above us a pigeon startles at the noise of my voice and flutters, battering its head on the glass stairwell roof. In the well below us lies a sodden old mattress half-covered by clots of grey feathers.

'It's a continual effort – to try to remember the humanity of the people that you're interacting with, and imagine what it is that makes their lives what they are, and makes them do what they do, particularly if they're being horrible to you. You're lifting against gravity, all the time. This kind of caring: it's effortful, at least for me. You can do this one.'

The doorbell isn't working. I knock hard, twice, a deep throated dog howls inside and we both take a step or two back into the shadows. There is a fiddling on a latch, a scratching of claws upon wood, a strangled kind of growl, and the door opens and a voice snarls, 'What time do you call this? We called *three hours* ago!'

Debbie's man stands braced, left hand twisted through the collar of a bullet-shaped dog which stands on its hind legs and is asphyxiating, pawing at the air between us, snapping and whining at the same time. The air is thick with stale weed and laundry.

'Nice dog!' says Theo, focused 100 per cent on the dog. 'What's he called then? Hey! Nice boy!' Theo crouches, the dog simpers and sinks to the floor, wagging the stub of its tail.

'Bullet,' says Debbie's man, disarmed. The chorus inside cries, 'Is that the doctor?' and Theo says, 'That'll be Debbie…' Her man sparks up again and says, 'She cannae fucking walk!

She's in agony! Three hours!' and Theo says, 'Yeah, busy, busy day, you know how it is … Great that you hung on though, and thanks for being so understanding, yeah?' Debbie's man, disorientated, says, 'Ah yeah, okay, thanks for coming, Doc… she's through here.' He lets loose the dog's collar and shambles down the corridor followed by Theo. I ease my way past the enchanted Bullet, who has now fallen dead asleep in the hallway.

Debbie is in a bad place. She lies in semi darkness on a couch, illuminated by flickering primary colours from a large screen bolted to the wall opposite as the sound system plays a revving of engines and a cycling beat-box rhythm accompanying a screen view of trucks hurtling through a winter vortex of highway. Debbie has, indeed, been peeing into a bucket, the odour of which is obscured by the smell of weed rising from the ashtray propped on the couch end.

'Hi, Debbie! I'm Theo Irvine. I'm Dr Dorward's student! Shall we move this, eh?' he says crouching to pick up the bucket, 'and this?', picking up the bowl of meaty doggie slurry beside it. 'Let's put it…'

'I'll take it,' says Debbie's man, now tame as his dog.

'Is that "Ice Trucker 4"?' asks Theo, taking the telly remote and curing my gathering migraine with one deft finger flick.

'What's happened then, Debbie?' he says, crouched by the couch, having taken her hand, ostensibly to check her pulse, but really just to take her hand. That magic, ancient, healing touch, the hand held, warmth exchanged, skin on skin, a finger on the pulse. When we lose these tiny skills, we lose everything.

'I just woke up, and I can't move my leg. It's agony. Electric shocks, all the way down the front, and numb too…'

'And when she tries to stand she just falls over. It's like her knee just gives way,' says her man.

'Did you hurt it?'

Slight, telling pause.

'No.'

'May I see?'

I switch the light on overhead but someone has installed a blue bulb in the socket and the shadowed blue gloom it casts is almost worse than no light at all.

Debbie is skinny and pale with thin red hair and Bic tatts on her knuckles with the names of two children who aren't anywhere to be seen, and as she shimmies out of her jeans I see skin covered in bruises and little sores. Her man shuffles, furtive in the background.

'Can I touch?'

Debbie whimpers her assent, and Theo moves her leg: flexes her hips, her knees, her ankles, squeezes her calf to find a clot, but there is nothing.

'Can you bend your leg?' She bends her leg. 'Can you straighten your leg?' Nothing. 'Can you flex your ankle?' She flexes her ankle. 'Can you push it up against my hand?' Nothing. Theo holds out his hand like a surgeon for a scalpel and I pass him a weighted tendon hammer. He taps her knee. Nothing. He taps her Achilles tendon, which twitches, gratifyingly.

'Can I just have a wee feel of your groin, Debbie?' She snuffles and nods. He feels. She yelps, snatches at his hand.

'Let me just have a wee feel, Debbie,' he asks, using the kind of soft voice you might to soothe a child. 'There's quite a big bruise in there, Debbie. I think it's pressing on the nerve.'

There's a bit of a pause. Her man stands with his hands in his pockets, looking at the floor. Bullet stands watching, repulsive stubby little tail cocked in anticipation.

'Might someone have jabbed something in there? A needle maybe?'

'Maybe...'

'I think you may have hit the nerve. By mistake.'

'It was him,' she mutters, under her breath. The man and his dog shrug their shoulders.

'You've bruised the nerve. It should get better when the swelling goes down. Might take a week or two, isn't that right?' He looks at me, for confirmation – being a student after all – and I nod.

'Should do.'

'So it'll get better?' says Debbie.

'Should do. But you'll need a lot of looking after. I guess he'll be doing a lot of running around after you. For weeks. Weeks and weeks. Everything you need…' Theo snaps his fingers. 'He'll bring it for you. Peeled grapes. Chocolate. Cups of tea. Anything you ask. Cos he's that sorry…' Theo stands, facing Debbie's man, whatever he is, passes a smile between them, one to the other, and under the clear light of Theo's smile, Debbie's man cracks one too. 'He's that sorry, Debbie, he's going to look after you, hand and foot…'

'Aye, that'll be right…' says Debbie, giggling a little now. 'And Ah want a foot massage too!'

'Aye! I will!' protests her man.

'*And* you'll be careful too, not to jag again, and if you do have to jag, you'll not jag there, because there's a lot of traffic goes that way, up and down your leg, and next time you might hit something serious, yeah?'

Debbie and her man nod their heads. *Wise words. Very wise.*

'And if it doesn't get better, though I'm sure it will, let us know?'

He stands to leave. Everyone's smiling now, even Bullet. 'Hey Boy!' says Theo as he passes, and Bullet's tail just can't help itself: it's off again, wagging.

'And,' he says, as if it is an afterthought, but really it's the thing that matters most of all, 'if the heroin thing, you know, the drugs, if they're becoming a bit of a problem, we're really happy to talk about that too you know. Just make an appointment. Dr Dorward here, he'll be really happy to help you with that...'

Their faces fall a little at this last.

'But can we not see *you* again, Dr Irvine?'

'Whatever it is, Theo, this thing that we've been trying to talk about – this *how to be good* – it's practical in its application. It's not just a theory. It takes a lot of skill to do it, and time and effort to acquire that skill.'

'It involves being decent to people. Kind, but in a practical kind of way,' says Theo.

'Most of the time. It's not respectful to be nice to people if they're not deserving of it. That's just patronising. We're not talking about mere *niceness* here.'

'Okay. But you still have to be *motivated* by a sort of kindness.'

'Generosity of spirit?' I say.

'And bravery,' says Theo. 'You have to be really brave. You have to be prepared to *take things on.*'

'And *see them through.*'

'And *take the consequences!*'

'That too.'

Theo pauses, thinks, says: 'It takes effort. And a *lot* of time.'

'But it's quicker in the long run. I think it wastes less time.'

'It's mysterious.'

'Perhaps. But people like you, *religious* people, use words like *mysterious* to cover up when they don't know what they're talking about, or when there is nothing *to* talk about. Bad habit, prevalent amongst believers. We need to keep this grounded.'

'Fair enough,' says Theo, who seems quite immune to offence, 'But you need to be okay in yourself too. It's really hard if you're not. You need good mental health. In fact, it's a *sign* of good mental health.'

'Unless it's obsessive. Some of the sickest people I've ever heard of have been saints.'

'Look at Saint Ursula.'

'What happened to Saint Ursula?'

'She was beheaded for refusing to copulate with the invading Huns.'

'Look at St Joan... Think of hair-skin shirts. Think of Thomas More. All that penitence and self-flagellation. And Mother Teresa...'

'Disagree with you there. You've just got a thing about Mother Teresa. She was okay.'

'Hmm. Don't agree. *I* think she was malignant and conceited.' I do, too, it's true. I can't find it in myself to like Mother Teresa.

'Which just goes to show,' says Theo, 'how little you know or understand. Whatever it is, it's merciful, and it's tolerant.'

'It gives the benefit of the doubt.'

'Without letting anyone take the piss. If you have it, you're no one's fool.'

'It's flexible. It's not dogmatic. It's intelligent, skilled and multi-faceted.'

'... doesn't moan and bitch all the time about the bad, but celebrates what's good...'

'Sounds like you're quoting Saint Paul.'

'Nothing wrong with that!'

'Quite a lot wrong with that actually ... The thing is, whatever it is, it's both the means and the end. It's the thing that is aspired to, and the journey there. So it's circular and self realising.'

'It's its own route and destination.'

'Original and of itself. Autochthonous.'

'Nice word.'

'Not one that is much used.'

'Mercifully.'

'So what are we to call it?'

'*I* would call it God,' says Theo, 'because I believe in God. Or His love, at least.'

'That's not much help to me. That's actively off-putting to me.'

'Okay. It's about trying to be good. Doing your best, all things considered.'

'Too banal.'

'Merciful.'

'Too hierarchical. Judgemental. Legalistic. Wrong.'

'Mutually respectful of autonomy and agency?'

'Ponderous, ugly, unconvincing, pseudo-philosophical…'

'*Compassionate?*'

'*Jackpot!* Worst of all: pious yet empty-headed, both self-congratulating and self-aggrandising. A word needing to be banned if any word were to be banned.'

'So what *is* the word that you're looking for?'

'I don't know. I'm not sure if there is one. But I think that *you*, Theo, are naturally good at it. And would be, God or not. It's like a talent. It's worth looking after.'

'That's kind of you to say. But not true. I'm no better than anyone else, and in a lot of ways worse.'

'You Christians are always making grandiose claims for your own sinfulness. It's a repulsive kind of upside down conceit. You should just accept praise where it's due, and criticism too.'

'Okay. But I learned it all from you, Dr Dorward.'

'That's not true either…'

———

Now, back to the present.

'Okay, *Dr Irvine*,' I say, a little punchier than I intend. 'Just send her home if that's what you're going to do. And if you do,

I'll certainly visit her tomorrow. But the first thing I will do is have a conversation with her about whether she really needs to be on warfarin, because she doesn't, because it will probably kill her faster than her tumour. So I'm pretty sure we'll be stopping it. You could perhaps just cut out the middle man and ask her yourself.'

Whatever it is, it's never arrogant. It's never aggressive nor dismissive and it doesn't trade in ultimatums. It doesn't throw itself around, impose itself on others, nor does it seek to humiliate.

'Okay, Dr Dorward, you do whatever it is you have to do. Thanks a lot, you've been very helpful.' *Not!* 'Goodbye.'

To think he and I had such mutual respect. We were almost friends once.

———

'What a *prat*! He must have thought you were such an *ass*!' says Lizzie, a doctor of 18 months' standing, who offers me the right generational perspective.

'He must have hated you!' says Donald, her junior doctor boyfriend.

'It's such typical *GP* arrogance!' says Thomas, my critical friend, who spits out the word 'GP' as if it's an expletive.

I felt a little weighed down by my conversation from earlier that day and sought to share it with people who might understand. I wish I hadn't now. It's not going as I had expected. Not a lot of sympathy coming my way. We four have been out running together. It has been beautiful. The stars are out and there is a full harvest moon low on the horizon, lit up pink by the recently set sun. It is the first crisp evening of the autumn, and we are all rosy and cold and have diverted into the pub where we are sitting drinking beer and waiting for chips. It is the end of the day, the best time of the day, and a good time to think it all through once more.

'Maybe it wasn't even him! Maybe I imagined the whole thing. The person I knew just wasn't like that. He's certainly changed.'

'It happens to everyone,' says Lizzie. 'He's a *jobs monkey*.'

'A what?'

'He starts his shift at seven with a list of jobs to be done from the last shift. By the end of the day he's lucky if he's got through half of them. He spends his day chattering around in his cage with all the other monkeys.'

'And the boss he mentioned?' says Donald, 'The one who did the ward-round and took all the decisions? He probably doesn't even know who that was. Couldn't ask him even if he wanted to. It could have been three shifts ago. Lost in history.'

'He probably doesn't even know the patient that you were talking about. She's a name on a list. That's the thing. He's just passing on a message. He's never met her!'

'He's just doing his best, all things considered. But it doesn't matter whether he's the most caring, best, most Mahatma-esque doctor that was born, he can't be any better than the system allows. *You're* just getting in the way, just making things even worse. Probably making him even *more* depressed than he already is!'

But it's the previous comment that really sticks – that seems critically important: *He's never met the patient. He's not even met the person that we were talking about.*

I find Mrs Dalrymple much changed when I go to visit her the next morning. She is thin and a little jaundiced. She is paler, un-spirited, hollowed out, abandoned, as if she has been left out overnight like a child's toy in the garden. She is gazing out of her sitting room window on the expanse of earth where her primroses once flourished. She manages a watery smile and half lifts her stick to greet me. 'I feel like I've been left out in the rain,' she says, weakly. That's one of the things that elderly people seem to say, when they're sad and at an end: '... *left out in the rain.*'

'I've come about your medicines,' I say.

'Oh, aye...'

I'm not sure she really knows who I am. That's the hospital effect. A lot of elderly people become like this after a long stay as an in-patient. It seems as if they have left a part of themselves behind. Sometimes, often, it is never recovered.

'Where are you keeping your medicines?'

She shrugs. She says, vaguely, 'I think they're in a box in the kitchen. The carer does all that for me now.'

Her kitchen is clean, and empty. There is no food out, nor evidence of cooking, no reading matter, no clutter, nothing left lying around. There is a medicine box on the kitchen table, and an unused walking frame by the back door. It is as if the house has become used to being empty.

'I was looking for the medicines that stop your blood clotting. Can you remember? Your warfarin. You were on it when you were in hospital. It's to stop your blood clotting. Do you know where you keep them?'

She looks at me through narrowed eyes, struggling to connect. Then she smiles, remembering something. 'I think someone maybe asked me about that...' She smiles again. '... last night, in hospital...' She struggles to recollect, her attention flickering, on and off, then connecting once again. '... in the middle of the night. A lovely doctor came and found me, sat with me for ages. Irish chap, I don't think I'd met him before. But he was *lovely*. Kind. He wanted to talk about my medicines – asked me which ones I was taking and why. We stopped the blood ones. Didn't seem much sense in me taking them...'

The Real Karlo Pistazja

'He's not the *real* Karlo, Doctor. That's the thing. The real Karlo is a sweet boy. Such a sweet boy. This one? I don't know. Words … can't…'

Words … can't … do the work that she wants of them. They can't bear the weight of what it is she has to tell me.

And she crumples into herself. I hand Mrs Pistazja a hanky and she cries, full throated sobs. Mrs Pistazja sobs into a hanky for her lost child.

She is a plump lady in early middle age. She looks after herself. Well kept deep black hair in an expensive bob, a nicely cut dark grey suit, a gold crucifix sitting on her chest. She's dressed herself up specially to come to see me. Her husband sits just behind her left shoulder. He is almost silent, struggling to hold it together as his wife weeps. She is plump, he is thin, dressed in his own formal black suit with its worn cuffs and scorch marks. Funeral suit. He's snatched some time from the business to be with his wife for this appointment, it matters so much. He works every hour that God gives him – he wouldn't neglect his business for anything, almost. But Karlo matters to them, more than business, or money. More than anything. Their only child.

'When did you notice that something was wrong?'

'He stopped answering his phone last week. He phones every day usually. But I thought to myself, he's a grown-up. He don't need to call us every day. He needs his space, he's a man now. He stopped coming to work. Karlo's always had his sick days. But then he sent us this.'

She pauses. She looks at her husband, appealing for permission perhaps, but he simply shrugs his shoulders. She reaches into her handbag, pulls out her phone.

'This was yesterday.'

... you cunt, get your teeth OUT OF ME ...

I glimpse, before she scrolls down the text:

... burning it all out so that at least I can breathe again, fucking burning it ALL ... before she swipes to the next as if she is ashamed to let me see what her son has sent.

'And then this was this morning.'

... please help me mum, please come, please help ...

'He doesn't write like that. Karlo doesn't want for anything. He doesn't need to ask for help. I went round to his flat ...'

She is crying again; her husband nervously puts a hand on her shoulder, but she shakes his hand away, thrusts the mobile phone under my nose, and I read:

... cunt help helpy cunt cunt help ...

And she says, 'This just isn't Karlo! This isn't the *real* Karlo!'

It happens rarely – every few years and always unexpectedly. Always, it seems, when you have other things to do, but perhaps that's true of all events in life that change you – those days which mark themselves in memory. This morning I was contemplating a full clinic and extras. I was teaching Nadja, my trainee, at 12, I had a meeting with a pharmacy advisor at lunchtime, a clinic in the afternoon, and I secretly wanted to leave a little early so that I could play tennis with my son. I wasn't unhappy about this – it's quiet days that sap me – but nonetheless, I had no space in the day, no redundant moment. Rita Pistazja phoned at 8 a.m., the moment the phones went across, the earliest that she possibly could. There was a message for me: *Rita Pistazja phoned about son Karlo (dob 1/3/1995). Behaving really oddly, please call, seems urgent.*

It's always bad timing when it happens.

This is a story that recurs, but rarely, every few years, no more. Not enough for one to gain expertise and never enough for you to be confident about how to handle it. Never enough to remember for next time what it is that you're meant to be doing. But I knew the shape of what was coming. You know already, at the first moment, that this is going to be a day lived on the verge of chaos. I text my son to tell him to find himself another tennis partner and call Rita back.

I had met Karlo a few times over the years. Karlo has cystic fibrosis, a not-so-rare inherited condition that causes progressive lung and digestive damage. When I was a junior paediatrician, I looked after children with cystic fibrosis. They needed daily chest physio to help them to cough up the thick secretions that clogged up their lungs, regular antibiotics, intravenous or inhaled, and regular medication to enable them to digest their food. They were rewarding children to look after, but the work could be hard to bear. They always seemed spirited and brave children, yet deteriorated steadily, hopelessly, and would always die, tragically young. Treatment for cystic fibrosis has been transformed in the last 20 years by better antibiotics, more intensive treatment, and the possibility of heart-lung transplantation which has opened up the possibility of near normal life expectancy for them.

Karlo *was* a sweet boy. Although most of his specialist treatment was undertaken by our local children's hospital, I knew him quite well. He still came in with his mother with all the other more minor things: eczema, coughs and colds, acne as a young teenager. He was a timid, rather ghostly child, who always clung to his mother's hand. He would try to hide behind her in a way that seemed to me to be archaic, 19th century like, as if he could conceal himself from me behind her voluminous skirts. He was thin and sallow and coughed thick mucus which he spat into a fresh hanky that his mother always supplied for him. When he was born and the diagnosis was obvious within the first days, Rita had herself sterilised. Karlo was to be her only child. Karlo was to be her job, her life, her hope, her tragedy.

'You went round to his flat?'

Rita looks at the floor. Her eyes fill with tears. Her husband takes her hand, and this time she accepts it.

'He wouldn't let me in. I had to shout through the letter box. I shouted "Karlo, if you don't let me in, I'm calling the police," and then suddenly he just opened the door.'

I wait. I give her time to collect herself.

'It *stank* in there, Doctor! The heating was right up full, and it was like he hadn't washed for days. He'd broken his television and his computer! He loves his computer! And he'd written things on the walls ... He'd written these terrible things. *On the walls*!'

She shakes off her husband's hand, gripping tightly onto the golden cross that was dangling from her neck.

'I ask him why he's broken his computer, and he just shouted back at me. It wasn't Karlo. It just wasn't him. What's happened to him, Doctor? Where has he gone?'

I don't know, not really. It could be dozens of things. It could be nothing – but I doubt it. I've heard this story before, a few times over the years, and never yet has it had an innocent explanation.

'I need to see him. Could you persuade him to come up?'

She shakes her head.

'He'll never come. He says there's nothing wrong with him. I said that I was coming to see you, and he just said, "Why?" Then he swore at me. That was when I phoned.'

I fitted Rita and her husband in, in between patients. I'm running very late now. The most nuanced decisions, the hardest ones, with the greatest consequence attached, always seem to be taken under pressure.

'I need to get on. I need to see the rest of my patients. Then I think you and I should meet at Karlo's flat. Decide what to do there. Let's see if he'll speak with me.'

I work my way through those many other tasks and problems that face me this morning. My mind is focused on each and every task.

My mind drifts elsewhere…

… mostly preoccupied with this spectre of madness. That Karlo has become *psychotic*. That the quiet boy, the sick and timid child who used to hide behind his mother's skirts, who suffers from a severe, life-limiting genetic disorder, is doubly cursed. I fear that Karlo is possessed by madness. That he may be hearing voices, a pandemonium of chattering hostility that no one else hears. I fear that the borders of Karlo's mind have become unclear to him: that his computer or his television is talking to him, personally, or that he is talking to the world through them; that he is scrawling messages on his wall because he has a message to impart to that world, or that that world is imparting something to him so dreadful that he must surround himself with protective amulets or spells to ward them off and protect himself. I fear that he will be paranoid, that he will be sat in the centre of a web of delusion: plots and spells, sticky falsehoods that tighten and suffocate, hold him so tight in their grip that he can never shake himself free.

My mind elsewhere, I see two children with fevers.

I see a young man with smoking-related heart disease who is worried because he can't breathe and thinks that he will die.

The demon madness lurks shrieking in the road ahead and I fear it.

I see a young woman who needs the pill, and another young woman with a breast lump which I think is benign.

I see an old man, a retired professor who has early dementia, who gives me a bottle of fine wine which makes me question my integrity, but which I accept anyway.

What does it mean, anyway, to be 'mad'?

I see a nervous young Bangladeshi man with perianal warts who quivers with shame and can't or won't tell me how he came by them, and then a hirpling old woman with osteoarthritis of the hip.

And what is it to be sane?

Then I see a fat 40-year-old woman who might just have appendicitis, though probably doesn't, but I just can't tell, so I send her to hospital.

I see a tremulous alcoholic with a scar on his face who wants something to help him sleep, but it's the booze that's doing it, and there's nothing I can do to help, and I won't lie to him, and so he leaves, buried by life, yet unprotesting.

I see a child with a cold, and another with earache, and yet another with a fever, whose mother had phoned in, demanding to be seen as an emergency, who I feared might be really, really sick, but has nothing wrong at all.

And I'm thinking...

... that Karlo has developed schizophrenia. That he is psychotic, but neither knows nor accepts it. That he probably won't want treatment. He will be aggressive, or dangerous, or just sad and inert. I'm worried that I won't know what to do and I'll let down his mother, whose pain I am beholden to, whose pain is colouring all my thoughts. I'm worried that I won't know what to do. That's always a worry. There isn't a doctor in the world who doesn't suffer from *that* one.

I sign 40 prescriptions. I skim read 28 letters, and respond to some phone calls.

Schizophrenia stalks and feeds upon the young. It is shape-shifting, subtle and insidious in its presentation. By profoundly and permanently affecting the mechanics of thought, it changes what you are, in the very centre of your self. It is not a pain that is *felt*, it is a pain that one *becomes*. It is the disintegration, and then the loss of the self, and I think that there can be nothing more pitiful than that.

I had a boy come to see me once, years ago, who was a maths student. I had met him before, a couple of times. I hadn't warmed to him much. He'd always seemed to me a little petulant and aloof, though there's nothing so unusual about that. But that day he seemed changed. He sat in front of me in my surgery, staring at the floor, just shaking his head, unable to find the words to tell me what it was that was wrong. He was a good-looking boy, but he smelled bad. His tutor had asked him to come to see me because she was worried, and his fellow students were complaining. He was hostile, unkempt, and they were becoming afraid of him. I was worried too, but, other than his silence, could find nothing wrong with him. I asked him to come back to see me a week or so later, so that I could try to understand better what ailed him, but he never came, and I forgot him. I see a lot of people in a week. I heard nothing more of him for several months, until I had a message that his parents wanted to come to see me. They told me that he had killed himself a couple of weeks previously: late one night he'd stood on the railings of a motorway bridge, right by his parents' house, and waited for a lorry to come. They had no idea, not even the tiniest shred of an idea why he had done this. He left no note, just a squalid bedroom and a school book full of jotted, incoherent mathematical symbols. I thought that his parents might be angry with me, that they might blame me, because I was the last doctor that he had seen, and that I had failed him. I *did* fail him.

I was anxious as I welcomed them into my room, offered them tea, but they were just sad and mystified and lost as they told me about their boy's slow deterioration over many months. They told me about how he'd left college, taken to his room, grown his beard, stopped washing. He, once a loving child, a brilliant young man, a great student, became folded in upon himself, silent, unable or unwilling to say what troubled him; he couldn't tell what it was that was going on in his head. His parents were on a kind of pilgrimage of grief. They were trying to retrace his steps, to remake all of his contacts over the last few months of his life, to try to know their lost child better, to try to reconstruct what it was that he had experienced, what had possessed him and changed him so – but really they were no nearer. They were no closer to understanding the source of their son's pain.

I had another patient, a student from Korea. In the place where I then worked there were many students from the Far East, talented people sent over by wealthy governments or parents to study useful subjects. He seemed polite, earnest, keen to please, incredibly diligent, at least compared to British boys of the same age. He was very similar to hundreds and hundreds of people whom I had looked after. There was nothing to differentiate him from the others like him. But he changed, and sharply, over a matter of just a few weeks. This straight-down-the-line electronics chap, a straight-A scholar, became a shiftless muttering creature, who had barricaded himself in his student room, surrounding himself with parts of telephones and computers and electronic kit that he had stolen from the university and wired together. The warden of his student residence had been called because of the hot smell of solder that permeated the landing where his room was, and when the boy wouldn't answer he'd called for help.

He trusted me enough to let me in to his room. I found him sitting in the centre of the floor of his little student cabin, in a cave of unconnected electronic hardware, surrounded by sheets of A4 paper taped down on the carpet. He was constructing a diagram, an electronic engineer's circuit diagram, a mind map of his world and the interactions of the many forces arrayed in it. He started to talk me through it: a vast and interconnecting conspiracy drawn in fine pencil web, shapes marked with symbols connected by vectors of perforated lines and arrows, and a finely drawn Manga-style oriental boy sat hunched in its centre which was a representation of self, yet unclear from the diagram whether a prisoner, or the controlling spider twitching upon the ends of long wires with a fine, bony finger. Prisoner or mastermind? Both at the same time perhaps, but nonetheless, him.

He had trusted me enough to let me in. Perhaps he shouldn't have, because after an hour or two of talk in which he had alluded, eliptically, to the harm that he might unleash upon his student landlord unless certain unspecified conditions were met, I called, on a semi-constructed pretext, a psychiatrist and a social worker, and the police as back-up to escort him to the hospital. When he saw them all arrayed outside his door he had taken fright and made for the shuttered window to jump – from four storeys up – but had bounced off the safety glass and into the arms of the police, who had subdued him and led him off.

It is always a momentous thing, to be instrumental in depriving a person of their freedom, even if that person seems dangerously ill. I had sat on the floor with that boy for a long time. There was no clear end to what he was saying, and no beginning, and no limit to the connections that he could make between imagined things, and I had had to listen to him intently. I had felt that I had to be absolutely sure of what I was doing. It is a momentous thing to deprive a person of their freedom.

It had made no sense, this pattern that he was trying so hard to construe, to pattern again on his dormitory floor, for *me*. But to him it seemed that everything depended on making me understand *something*. He had looked at me through narrowed black eyes, forehead creased with concentration, so full of fear, trying so hard to *make me know too*. Nothing mattered more to him than that I listen and understand what that *thing* was. The boy he had previously been was in there still – lost and occluded, but there. I had glimpsed him, from time to time, tangled, bound head and foot in strong, imagined silk, lost in his web.

I have no doubt that in that case I acted well, that I saved his mind, possibly even his life – and that happens rarely in my line of work – but nonetheless, there was violence done to that person by me, when I called the police on him.

He came to see me a few weeks later. The boy I had known first, before he became ill, was snake thin, fit looking, eager, ready, vitally intelligent. Already now, just weeks into his illness, he was running to fat. He was ponderous, a little slow.

The antipsychotic that he had been prescribed, risperidone, does that. It changes your mind, changes your shape, changes the person you are. Yet, he was incomparably better. He just wanted a letter from me for his tutor to say that he was okay to study again. Tentatively, I asked after his mental health. Was he still hearing voices? Was he afraid of anyone, or anything? Did he have any special powers? Did he ever feel that things were sending messages – radio, television, the internet, his computer – directed at him personally? He shook his head, flushed a little with shame, said, 'No, Doctor, I'm *fine* now…' I asked about the spider web diagram that he had tried to talk me through, just a few weeks previously, during that long evening kneeling on the floor of his cabin, and he shuddered with embarrassment. He made the international nut-case gesture with his forefinger to his temple rotated clockwise thrice and said, 'Loop the loop, Doctor, loop the loop. I'm fine now,' and by then, certain enough that he was, I let him back to college.

Months after his diagnosis, he was studying again, but not so well. He had become, in his own terms, stupid. Months after his diagnosis, he had become tremendously overweight, and, never fat before, these rolls of flesh were unbearable to him. He felt himself wrapped within another person, in his own words, 'suffocated inside a jelly-roll'. He felt tired, and lazy; he had no new, good, original thoughts. Just months after his diagnosis, he wanted to stop his risperidone. 'This isn't me,' said the boy I had once known, calling out to me from deep within his pools of fat.

The invention of effective antipsychotics have both transformed the treatment of severe mental illness, the *psychoses,* and helped us to re-imagine what these illnesses might be. Since the development of chlorpromazine in the 1950s, diseases which were devastating to the brains of sufferers have been partly ameliorated.

Uncontrolled, florid psychosis has the effect of burning through the psyche. You don't stay incandescent like that, for very long. You burn out: incapable of volition, of thought, of experience, your brain becomes a fleck of ash. With burned-out schizophrenia you sit in a kind of mental darkness, rocking and muttering, quietened now behind your veil of suffering. You can remain like that for decades. You don't see that much, anymore, and that's because of the mind-saving effects of antipsychotics, probably.

But it doesn't feel like that if you are actually taking the drugs. People taking antipsychotics don't, by and large, feel grateful. Although the recollection of *being* psychotic can be a recollection of suffering – of terrible, pervasive fear, of being possessed, cut off from self, disrupted in a profound and terrifying way – being on antipsychotics brings with it its own, more subtle, deficits. Within the labyrinth of psychosis can echo something precious. Psychotic illness can exaggerate and distort certain parts of cognition which make us what we are, core elements of what makes us human and ways of being which are precious to us – the ability, for example, to think in an original and creative way. The capacity to make odd connections between disparate domains of thought. The ability to think of oneself as *other*, to imagine the voices of others in one's own head, and act on the instructions and volition of a person or a being which is conjured, or remembered, or simply imagined. Abilities that you can't imagine a machine having, or an animal, be it ever so intelligent. And it seems that the effect of antipsychotic medicine is, to a greater or lesser extent, to cut you off from these abilities. Sometimes, despite the horror and pain of the illness itself, the psychotic patient in remission will recollect that early period of their illness, that up-tic in sensibility, perception and cognition, and remember it almost with nostalgia, as the time when they felt most intensely alive.

This story, of a patient manifestly benefiting from a drug yet desperate to stop it, is a familiar one to psychiatrists. It can seem that whole benign, yet coercive, structures are maintained around these people to keep them on their meds.

So he wanted to stop his drugs. Deferential and respectful, however, he wouldn't, not without my say-so. A year or so in, he was failing at college, depressed, dishonoured by his community of fellow students. 'Now that I'm a fat and stupid person, I'm not a part of the crowd. There doesn't seem much point in going on,' he said to me matter-of-factly one day.

'With your course? With your life? What do you mean?'

'Just that. I'm not *me* anymore, and there's no point in what I've become.'

I consulted with his psychiatrist; we compromised on cutting his dose. I reviewed the boy every week, fearful of a resurgence, of the return of the manga boy twitching in his spider's web. He did transform, true, but in a good way. As if by some process of magic, within a few weeks, the person I had first known was returning. He shed his weight. He shed that other jelly-roll self and emerged like some long limbed agile creature basking under a new sun. His grades improved, his mood was transformed, he got a girlfriend, smiled a lot, admitted to me a little shamefaced one day that he had stopped his risperidone altogether. It had stopped him functioning properly sexually, and now he could. This mattered even more than his good grades, he confided, hiding a half smile and a blush. I continued to meet him once a week, but now it was more social really. Whenever I asked him how he was feeling, he would shrug and say, 'Great'. Whenever I asked him, as I occasionally did, about his web of conspiracy, he would look embarrassed, shudder again, in that way, and change the subject, so I stopped asking.

I left that job to go to another. But I did a thing with that patient I had never done before, nor since.

When I told him that I was leaving, he looked downcast. We had come to know one another well. A few weeks before I was due to move on, he came to see me, clearly troubled, clearly a little embarrassed. There was something that he wanted to ask me. I waited. Red faced and shy, he asked whether, now that I was leaving, it might be possible, in some way, that we be friends. Generally, I'm not open to friendships with people who are also patients. There are just a whole lot of reasons why it's easier that way. But for him, for cultural reasons, I think that asking me that question was very brave. I don't know this – I don't know anything about Korean culture, and perhaps I am making unwarranted assumptions, but that was what I thought at the time. I thought that this was an enormous, brave, cultural leap in the dark. So I hesitated before responding. *What would such a friendship look like?* or words to that effect.

'You play tennis…,' he said. There was a court by the car park opposite my practice. I used to play sometimes with Adam, the practice psychotherapist, at lunchtime. There was a racquet and balls propped in the corner of my room.

'I do…'

'So do I. Perhaps we could play?'

'Okay…' Then, tentatively, '… but tell me … why?'

'Because,' he said, struggling, reddening, 'because you … know me … *all* of me.'

We played a few times. I was stronger, he was far younger and fitter. He used to win, which I think he liked. I moved on. We met only a few times after that, and then lost contact.

***

At half past 11 I meet Rita outside Karlo's house. A block of flats in a nice enough area. Well-kept green space outside, clean windows, curtains open, all but one, in the corner of the ground floor, where thick yellow drapes are jammed shut and there's a pile of clothing on the ground outside the window. It's just Rita there. The father has gone back to work, I think, or feared to become involved. We go around the side and she knocks on the door, but there's no answer. She bids me hang back, raises her forefinger to me. She'd said that if he saw me, and knows that I'm there, he'd never open the door. He'd just pretend not to be in. I hang back. I don't like this – I don't like any kind of deception – but she knows best. She calls in through the letter flap: '*Coo-ee* Karlo, it's your mother...' and there is a stirring from deep inside the flat and the door opens, and she goes in, signalling as she does that I might follow.

'I brought the doctor with me.'

I stand in the hallway. The floor is thick with unopened mail, brochures, election fliers. White goods, a fridge and a washing machine, block the way. A nebuliser – a piece of medical equipment to help the boy breathe – stands unopened in packaging. It is hard to breathe. As his mother had said, it is hot. The heating is on full, the curtains are closed, and the smell of sweat and smoke – that scouring, animal odour – suffocates.

'What the fuck...!' he shouts at his mother, who flinches at his swearing, as if she has been hit.

'What the fuck do you call the doctor for, Ma?'

Karlo is not the boy I once knew. I see this immediately. I realise that I have been imagining a boy from time past, long previous, the boy of ten years ago, somehow unchanged. I was expecting some kind of doomed Victorian orphan child, having re-imagined him as a dark-clad phthitic mad wraith coughing blood, quivering in his sick bed.

Far from it. Karlo has muscled up. He stands bull-like in his cave, shags of black curly hair, grey vest and underpants. He's framed by the dark door to his sitting room, where I see the remnants of the television, broken electronic stuff, a mattress over the window, a bench press on the floor. Karlo has muscled up and the idea pops into my head: *anabolic steroids? Roid rage?*

'Why the fuck did you call the doctor? You had no right to call the doctor!'

The tone of his speech is loud, flat, unvarying, bull-like. He bellows. He is sweating, his chest is pumped out, his head thrust forward, he snorts and shows his teeth. There's prey enough left in my DNA for me to read the signs. He's ready to charge. I hang back.

But Rita has no fear. This is her son, after all. She marches up to him and jabs a finger in his chest and says, 'You don't speak like that in front of a doctor, Karlo!' and then to me, 'Come in, Doctor. Karlo doesn't mean it. He's a good boy.' And so I take a step forward.

Karlo does mean it though. Karlo blunders forward, pushing his mother out of the way, and shouts, 'You're not coming in! Fuck off! Get back!' Karlo is breathing fast, sweating, angry, fearful. Karlo is casting around for a weapon. I take a step back.

But then Karlo stops for a moment. He thinks. Karlo restrains himself. It is as if some previous Karlo, his slower, better self, interposes between the raging minotaur Karlo and myself. Says, more calmly, 'I'm telling you to leave. If you don't leave right now, I'm calling the police.'

Karlo is suppressing his rage. Karlo is calculating. Something in Karlo, some other part, is exerting control, suppressing whatever beast it is that makes him snort and paw the ground. Whatever: the dynamic has altered, there has been a change of pace and the threat is dissipating. Karlo says, 'I'll come and see you, Doctor. okay?' He even manages a little half smile at this point.

Rita, who wants action, wants this problem dealt with, and who can blame her? She sees my uncertainty, and I can see her disappointment. But Karlo is right. Or so I think. I don't *know*. But right now, I think, why *am* I not just a housebreaker? It's me that's the intruder. I have no right to be there. If I were in America, he could shoot me dead, and no one would criticise him. The police get called and it's me that'll be cuffed, or so I think. I haven't checked. I don't *really* know.

'Okay,' I say, and Rita's face falls. 'I'll see you in an hour. I'll see you at my surgery in an hour. I'll have plenty of time then, and we can talk. I'll see you then, okay?'

Slowly, slowly, I back off.

I don't really expect him to show up. This is time bought: to retrench, retreat, gather my forces. I have used the Mental Health Act as a means of compulsorily admitting and treating a patient against their will about five times in the last 25 years. I remember the face of each patient whom I have perpetrated this thing upon. The act is long and complex, but the gist is simple: If someone has a *mental illness* of a certain pre-determined and arbitrary kind, and they are an immediate, urgent risk to themself or to someone else, and they absolutely refuse assessment, and there is no less restrict-ive way of managing the situation, then you consult with a social worker who is the designated duty Mental Health Officer, and fill out a long-ish form, and call the police and an ambulance. Then call whoever it is that you have at home and tell them not to wait up for you. You will be late. It is your job to ensure the person is safe and alive when they get to hospital. If you break a thing, you have to fix it. It feels a terrible thing to impose your will on another – to take away their freedom, however sick or mad they may be.

Everything hangs, however, on what is meant by *illness*, defined as '*mental illness, personality disorder or learning disability, however caused or manifest…'* It doesn't count, though, if you are drunk or intoxicated with drugs. It doesn't count if you are simply being very, very *imprudent*, as the act quaintly states, no matter how imprudent. It doesn't count if your ailment is a non-standard sexuality, even if that sexuality is very unappealing, or even criminal. 'Personality disorder' covers a very wide range of possibilities indeed, and any of the above exceptions might be a *symptom* of an underlying mental disorder in any case. So confronted with the problem, as I am, the weapons of state that I have to hand – legal, medical, definitional – are indeterminate. They seem strangely blunt and soft.

I call the psychiatric hospital for advice. I ask to speak to the duty psychiatrist, but am repeatedly put through to a young sounding doctor who I think just happens to be standing by the phone. She is very nice, but she sounds about the same age as my god-daughter, and knows less about the relevant provisions of the mental health act than I do. I call the social work department and ask for the mental health officer and leave a message for her to call me back. Leaving messages for the social work department can feel like you are hefting a large stone down a very deep well. I try to look up the provisions of the act on Google, but my NHS desk computer freezes. Finally I am reduced to my smartphone: squinting into a tiny screen, pecking at the keys like a schoolchild.

An hour later, to my surprise, Karlo turns up. He seems less imposing now that he is dressed, now that he is on *my* territory. Courtesy of my smartphone, I am boned up on the relevant provisions of the Mental Health Act. Now I feel confident. 'Emergency Detention Order': these were the words I had been struggling to recollect. I have printed off the right form that I need to fill. It's sitting there, ready on the desk, ready to go.

He comes in and sits. He posts a fake smile; it makes him look shady. He shakes a little in his chair. In the better light of my office, I can see that his lips are blue. He is cyanosed, we say, a cardinal and sinister feature of the heart/lung disorder that will kill him if his mental disorder doesn't do the job first. He smells of smoke, and he is breathless. When I used to work with kids with cystic fibrosis, they always used to start smoking, at the age of 14 or so. In the unit, it felt like a family bereavement. It brings your death on by a decade or more – that's 50 per cent if you're a 'cystic'. Karlo is far sicker than he needs to be. He hasn't taken his medication for months. His prescriptions have lain unclaimed, and no one has noticed. He stares at me, still smiling – mouth smile, no eyes.

'So why do you have to see me so urgently?'

Always be honest.

'Your mother is really worried about you, and so am I. I'm worried that you might have developed an illness that's making you upset and behave oddly. I'm worried that you might not be taking your medication because of it. You could die without your medication.'

He laughs. His laugh is empty of emotional content. As is his smile.

'Do you think I've got a *mental disorder*?'

His use of the words 'mental disorder' strikes me as odd.

I ask him questions: 'Can you hear voices that others can't? Do you have any special powers? Do you feel that there is some kind of plot directed against you?' But increasingly my questions feel forced and artificial. He wears that painted smile, laughs that empty laugh and says, 'No, no and no.'

I confront him with the texts that he sent to his mother, and he laughs again, and I wish that he would stop. He says, 'There's an explanation for that....,' and I say, 'What?'

It feels as if we are each enacting roles. Going through a performance. Neither of us has any faith in what we are saying.

'I was acting as a consequence of my use of *intoxicating drugs*.'

In real life nobody speaks like this.

'What drugs?'

He shrugs his shoulders. He actually shrugs his shoulders. I want to hit him.

'Cocaine. Speed.'

I have this very strong sense that, whilst I was sitting in my surgery Googling the provisions of the Mental Health Act (Scotland) 2003, Karlo was doing exactly the same thing. I have this very strong sense that he's quoting the Mental Health Act at me.

'Right. Do you use a lot of ... cocaine?'

'No. Just this weekend.'

'Why are you smoking? Why haven't you been taking your medication?'

'Because I'm being very *imprudent*.'

Now he's taking the piss. The smile's still there – but it's no longer totally empty. It is a little impish. One version of Karlo, real or not I don't know, knows now that he's *winning*.

I wait, thinking over the next best step. Hope of any kind of resolution dissipates rapidly. I wish I'd opened the windows. It is a hot day, and the boy still hasn't showered. His clothes are filthy. You can't send someone to a locked ward for not washing. You can't send someone to a locked ward for smoking themselves to death, however young they are. You can't send someone to a locked ward for taking drugs.

I keep in my room stacks of saliva testing kits for intoxicants. They test for cocaine and stimulants. I suggest it.

'Why? I've already told you I've been doing coke...' But, indifferent, he takes the swab anyway, pops it in his mouth, and chews it.

I suggest that he might like to see someone at the hospital to offer a second opinion. He doesn't see the point, but he's not much bothered. He knows the pressure's off. He shrugs his shoulders again, agrees to go. I phone the nurse at the mental health assessment service, tell him about this guy I'm really worried about, with late stage cystic fibrosis, not taking his meds, mother thinks he's behaving really oddly, could all be drug induced but I think he's probably psychotic, but pretending not. The nurse is calm and reassuring as I recount the story. Unlike me, he deals with this kind of crisis every day.

'Sure,' he says, 'send him up. I'll see him. Don't hold your breath though.'

Let me ask you. What makes you the *real* you?

When I was a child of five or six, my brother and I used to stay for long weekends with two elderly aunts who stayed in a town a few hours drive from where our parents lived. The distance felt remote. They had no telephone, their house was cold, heated by a single coal fire which needed to be cleaned out and raked, built anew every morning, stoked up into a fierce friendly glow by the afternoon. They lived in a different time: nothing in the house, or their clothes, or their language, or the food they ate, dated beyond the thirties. When our parents drove away, we could feel the decades settling over our heads, the muffling strata of ages.

They were loving. They had high, very particular, expectations of us. Nessie, the older of the two, had been a school teacher, and expected us to read to her in the evenings from Edwardian cautionary tales with names like 'Little Johnie Head in Air'. We read. We ate home-made tomato soup and porridge. We trod the house softly and spoke with muffled voices and played as children of the thirties would have played, as we imagined our father with his brothers had done, and used their imagined voices, and their words and manners, as if we were two ghosts.

'I *say*, Andrew!'

'Yes, *old sport?*'

'Shall we play cricket?'

Wrapped as we were for a couple of days in their world, we assimilated. Without a thought, we became *of* their world. We couldn't have done otherwise.

Nessie and her sister Jorrie, who did all of the driving, used to take us in the afternoons, to visit their round of deserving elderly: a distant aunt jilted in love who had taken to her bed in 1942 and hadn't got up; her dementing older sister; a blind old man with half a jaw who was fed from a spoon, who choked and coughed when he tried to talk, and sprayed forth his tea and scone across a rubberised bib which Nessie mopped down after with a special little towel she'd brought with her packed in a reticule. Andrew and I were silent, cowed by all this lurking horror.

One afternoon they took us to visit two very old women and the man that lived with them. The women were, I think, demented, or at least, as they say now, cognitively impaired, and are greyish ghosts in my memory: two hunched figures sitting at a heavy table in a cluttered parlour while the old man served tea from a silver service, plopped in sugar lumps with a pair of silver tongs and asked Nessie in song-like Scots whether '*the bairns wid have a wee dab o' jeelie on their piece?*' His hair was oiled and white and combed back into a ruthless parting, and he wore a navy blue gabardine suit with a silver watch chain. He *flirted* with my aunts. His face was smooth and pink, the plumped skin laced with fine wrinkles. As we were getting in the car after, Nessie said, 'Jorrie, isn't it *odd*!'

Heavily bored until then, Andrew and I spark back into awareness, wondering what could possibly be *odd*.

'What's odd, Nessie?'

'Isn't it odd how *Agnes* is getting more and more like a *man*!'

The shocked little boys sat in the back of their aunties' car, scrabbling to reassemble the shards of a world whose crystalline certainty was shattered.

If you can't rely on something as stable as the gender identity of your great-aunties' friends, what is there left that's solid in the world?

Lacking the vocabulary, however, and being somewhat repressed, we didn't discuss it for *years*.

These two shocked boys are as remote from us now as characters from history or fiction. The aunts are long since dead, the identity of their gender pioneering friend utterly un-recoverable.

'Did I remember this right?' I asked, over beer, in front of friends, years later, and Andrew said, 'Yes! Do you remember her hair? Do you remember her blue suit, the watch-chain and her pink skin?'

'Do you remember, "Nessie, isn't Agnes getting more and more like a *man*?"'

Everyone laughs: everyone enjoys Andrew's falsetto imitation of the aunties' recollected voices.

'But which of the aunts was it that actually *said* that?'

The memory has been passed between us, countless times, over decades. Because it's funny. Because it's safely shocking, even now. Because it raises questions about identity, gender, and memory: questions that don't go away.

It's a shared memory, down to its tiniest details; we share the tiniest details, Andrew and I. Which of these details are original to me, and which to Andrew, I couldn't say. I *know* the truth of the story though, because the memory is vividly mine: I can *see* his/her pink lined face, now, in my mind's eye, though I wouldn't swear that she was really called Agnes. It might have been Mary.

What makes a thing still the same thing over time? And what makes a person so? And which version of the countless persons we can be in our lives is the *real* person? And which of those countless impulses that assails me in a single instant is *me?* And why might one matter more than any of the others?

According to Locke in *Identity and Diversity*, a person is 'a thinking intelligent being, that has reason and reflection, and considers itself as itself, the same thinking thing, at different times and places.'

Locke had a purpose. Writing in 1689 after decades of civil war and religious intolerance, he sought to construct a political philosophy founded not so much on the rights of monarchs, or the contestable diktats of churches or different versions of God, but on the rights of individuals. Locke needed strength, flexibility, resilience in his theory of personhood if it was to serve as his foundation stone. His conception of personhood and personal identity was necessarily *forensic* in its nature: it had to provide binary answers to binary questions. *When does a person begin and end? When does a person matter? When does a person's responsibility begin and end?* Locke *needed* a theory of stable personal identity, and he provided one: so successfully that his conception of personhood forms the basis of how the law sees us now, and how we see the law; it works so well, that it provides the basis for how we see ourselves. But a person is a thing that remembers. Everything depends on memory, and these luminous moments of awareness are unreliably recollected. A person assembles a chain of such recollection, which disappears back, losing itself into the mist of *before*. A person is like a necklace: different coloured beads of awareness, randomly selected, strung on a thread of memory.

I don't know which of my memories of Agnes are mine, and which are Andrew's. I know that some of them are real, some constructed, some imagined, some started life as elaborations on a good story. I experience them all nonetheless just the same, as *mine*. I fear that the Agnes transsexual paradox might raise questions which are fatal to my theory of self. I fear that a lot of my memories, impulses, ideas, experiences are susceptible to the same kinds of objections: they're not *really mine*, they're just there.

The philosopher Derek Parfit is famously skeptical about our ordinary assumptions about self-hood and identity. He uses appealing thought experiments involving minds that can divide, or minds that can fuse, or the idea of networks of branching and re-uniting selves with shared memories which are *real* but strictly unattributable, and he calls these q-memories, and describes the intentions of those people whose characters are formed of these q-memories as q-intentions. I find my experience better described by Parfit than Locke. He is a gentle writer. He implies that the question of personal identity only really matters for forensic or legal reasons. That without those imperatives, the question no longer demands a yes/no response. Identity becomes a matter of degree, something that can come and go, a thing dependent on *context*.

In his book *Don't Sleep, There are Snakes*, the linguistic philosopher and former missionary, Daniel Everett, describes a lifetime working among an Amazonian tribe, the Pirahã. The Pirahã are described as having no material culture, no symbolic culture and no concept of a world beyond that of immediate experience. Their unique language is simpler in terms of vowels and phonemes than almost any other, yet hardest to learn. It is an expression of their culture – to learn the language is to learn the culture, and the two are inseparable. It has no capacity for a past and future tense, and pronouns are a recent borrowing. The Pirahā have the weakest possible grasp of personal identity and responsibility, and no moral theory beyond their immediate responses. A person disappearing around the bend in the river in his canoe is not necessarily the same person who returns that evening with fish. Dreams aren't distinguished from lived life, and the world of spirits are undistinguished from that of solid things. People change their names and their selves, and memory and experience are shared.

Everett and his theories have been attacked. As practically the only non-native speaker of a rapidly disappearing language, they are hard to test. He writes with compassion; his own identity, faced with the intellectual and cultural challenge posed by the Pirahā, becomes porous. He loses his religious faith; his whole world view is overturned by the lived example of the civilisation he had sought to convert. The world he describes is more Parfit than Locke.

It only takes one counter-example to bring down a theory.

But none of the above is helping with the immediate problem that's troubling *me*. Which is this: that, all other things being equal, we must respect the autonomy of persons – that's a core value in our society. *I* think that it should be a core value in *all* societies. But we don't respect the autonomy of certain kinds of persons whose mental function is transiently disturbed by reason of certain kinds of mental illness, even though they might continue to have memory, reason, awareness and identity sufficient to satisfy Locke's criteria. Sometimes we detain them on locked wards. Sometimes we *impose* treatments on them, change them to the core, sometimes to protect others, but often, to protect a future, preferred version of themselves. It's as if, behind Locke's forensic idea of personhood, we have another (ghost) theory, which entails the concept of a *real,* most legitimate version of a person, whose autonomy must be respected most of all. And then, by implication, progressively less real, less legitimate versions, whose autonomy can be respected less. But I don't understand what, in this instance, we can possibly mean by *real*.

So Locke's theory of personal identity doesn't help me much with Karlo and his mother.

'He's just not the *real* Karlo anymore, Doctor…'

The nurse in the psychiatric unit lets Karlo go – and I think he's right to. He phones me later in the afternoon and explains: yes, he shares my worry. There is obviously something not right, but nothing, as he puts it, that we can hang a diagnosis on. He might be 'prodromal' – in the early stages of a psychotic breakdown, but not sick enough, yet, to treat compulsorily. It might all just be the drugs he's taking, and he's allowed to do that. I agree with the nurse. If Karlo were in pain with his symptoms, if he were suffering the kind of mental torture that you see commonly with psychotic or depressed people who lack insight, then I can see the justification for treating him compulsorily. Or if he were threatening another person, it would be easy, comparatively. But I think, by and large, that Karlo should be permitted to take all the drugs he wants, and all the alcohol too, even if that's going to kill him, however *imprudent* I believe him to be – to think otherwise is futile, and illiberal. He'll just go on and do it anyway. A different part of me, however, thinks that that is absolutely nuts. He's just a child of 25, he doesn't know what he's doing. He's someone's son – I have sons, I know what they can be like – and he's going to die soon. Something needs to be done.

The saliva swab comes back negative. No cocaine, no amphetamines, not even marijuana, which is rare for this demographic. I confront him. I phone him up – I beg him, practically, to come back to see me. I have spoken with his chest physician. At his last check-up his heart/lung failure was dire. He is comparatively free of symptoms at present, but he is teetering. He turns up a couple of weeks later.

'Your saliva sample was negative.' I wait for a response. He smiles. He's shaved his head. All those curls are gone. He has a tattoo behind his left ear, intruding onto his cheek, which I think may be new. A paw of some kind, with blooded claws. I don't look too closely. His mother will be heartbroken. He reeks of cigarettes and sweat.

'What's with the spit sample? Why did you lie to me?'

That same unvarying, emotionally dead smile.

'You were going to send me into hospital. I have stuff to do.'

'What stuff.'

He shrugs. 'Stuff online. Just stuff.'

Okay.

I lost touch with Karlo. It was a few years ago, and I fear now that he might be dead.

Sometimes I imagine alternative histories for myself – how things might have turned out different. What would have happened to me, say, if I had actually *passed* that exam? Or attempted that scary jump when I was 15, or practised harder or better on the violin, or got in that car with that man when I was a child? I think we all probably have those *what if* thoughts, some bringing comfort, some an odd kind of speculative pain.

Sometimes I wonder about Karlo. What if he *hadn't* taken those mind altering drugs I'd supposed he had? What if he had listened better to his mother, or to me? What if he had accepted treatment? What if he had grown to be the young man his parents had wanted? What if he had studied, never got that life-changing facial tattoo? What if he had got his transplant, had a normal kind of life? What if he had inherited the business that his father had built for him? All idle stuff really. Dreams, stories, imagination, nothing. Karlo took his own path, made his own choices. That was the one *I* knew: *that* was the real Karlo.

The Words to Say It

‘You said it! These were *your* words!’

‘I … But…!’

I didn't!

‘You said: "It's all in your head!"’

I couldn't! I wouldn't have! You see, I *know* this. Because I have never said that to a person. Even when I have been thinking exactly that: *It's all in your head!* I have never mouthed that thought.

‘But … but…’

But I can't finish the sentence. Even now I can't find the words to say it.

Antonio sits forward at the table. Pinning me with those piercing blue eyes of his. His mum and dad sit on each side of him. On my right is Dr Suarez, his neurologist, and on her right is Julie, a urology nurse. On my left is Dr Morgan, his psychiatrist, and on her left is Dr Craig, an interventional radiologist. An airless little conference room set just off a hospital ward, and it's seven adults ranged against young Antonio, who sits leaning forward, staring at me through narrowed, angry eyes, and says, ‘I used to trust you. But that's what you said. These were *exactly* your words. You told me that I was just making it all up.’ And not for the first time I think *how powerful this child is!* Antonio was 15 then.

'… I'm sorry,' I say, at last. 'That wasn't what I meant.'

'But it's what you *said*.'

I have known Antonio since he was little. He is a treasured only child. His father is a maths teacher, and his mother teaches piano at a private primary school.

It was with me – under my care at least – that things started to go wrong.

Antonio was a special kind of child. Everyone described him that way. His parents are brown eyed, but Antonio's are a piercing violet blue. His father blinks through thick glasses shambling and stumbling through a complex, difficult world strewn with obstacles; young Antonio skipped through his with tiny light velvet-clad feet. His mother is overweight and though only 40, limps with a stick; Antonio is long and supple limbed. When talking, when distracted, he stretches, ballet dancer's stretches: he stands on one foot, grips the opposite toe between thumb and forefinger, stands straight backed, lifts his other foot like a new branch on a sapling tree, carries on talking. Showing off? Probably. He has thick red hair which he keeps from his eyes with an equine toss of his head. There is, was, something animal-like, something of the thoroughbred, about that boy.

His parents aren't wealthy. He goes to an ordinary school, half a mile or so from my office. The others in his year might as well be of another species: the mortal human species perhaps. Other boys his age are just growing thin beards, faces speckled with sores, voices booming as they jostle to be first. Of them, some of the thin ones still play football, still leap around, untamed in the wild world, but half of them have migrated already to games consoles, languishing. Antonio is not like that. Antonio has always been different. It is as if he is of another kind. He loved to perform. As a nine-year-old, he won competitions in tap dance. A wee kilty boy with red hair and a blur of feet, rattling and tapping and leaping higher than any of the other children; straighter backed, he seemed to hang in space longer than would seem possible for a mortal body. At 10 he had moved to Theatre and Mime, at first a weekend theatre school in Glasgow, but latterly he had had sniffs from others – conservatoires: London, Birmingham, *Paris*...

He had always seemed full of confidence. As far as I could tell, he wasn't unhappy. Despite his anomalous type, he wasn't bullied. He was excited to be going. This world here was clearly no place for Antonio. There was no space for him. It was too small, the species pool was too limited, there was no one else here like him. London would be different. Paris even more so. He already had quite good French, picked up on holidays with an aunt in Bordeaux and from a passion he had for old-style French pop. *Avec le temps, toutes s'en va*... Unguarded, he used to sing under his breath. He was an unusual boy.

Back then, back before things started to go awry, Antonio was mainly in the slipstream of my attention. It was his mother that occupied me most. While the boy, the child, had flickered and danced and stretched and played on the floor, his mother would tell me about her illnesses. Her life has been blighted by illness. Tiredness. Pain. Guts. Joints. Skin. Bladder. Tiredness.

She had once, she says, been full of promise too, glancing from the corner of her eye at her flame-haired child playing in the corner, pretending to be a cat, stalking a mouse. Antonio must be about five. Four or five. *She* had been a high achiever too. She had been a piano student at the Royal Academy in London, but had developed unexplained neck and forearm pain which had snuffed out her potential.

I see the boy, out of the corner of my eye, pounce upon a scrap of paper lying under my couch. For a moment, for an instant, he *is* a cat.

'But it didn't matter in the end. I met this one's father...' She rolls her eyes, assuming that I will understand exactly what is so bad about *that*. '... and then I was pregnant.' She pauses, shifts her weight in the chair, makes the 'Ooof' sound, that people make when they need to show, in a quiet kind of way, that they have pain. She moves her stick a little, prompting me, reminding me: she walks with a stick. She has pain.

'And then you got ill...'

'Well, I thought that it was just normal tiredness, with pregnancy, sleepless nights, feeding and so on. But that didn't explain the *pain...*'

'No,' I say, feeling within myself the ghost of her tiredness, some pain.

'And that was when *you* missed the diagnosis.'

Antonio, bored now, tugs at his mother's elbow, and she pats his hand, a little briskly, and says, 'Not now, Toni.'

'Well...' I say, also becoming a little irritated with Antonio, who immediately desists, finds the toy box I keep in the corner and rattles through it.

'Well...' I say, but we have been through this about a thousand times before. Antonio's mum had a very slightly abnormal blood test a few years previously: borderline raised *antinuclear antibodies*. The test is positive in cases of Lupus, which is a serious connective tissue disease, which can cause, among other much worse things, tiredness, depression, and joint pain. The blood test, though, is hopeless as a screening test, because it's often positive in the normal population, who very often indeed suffer from non-specific symptoms of tiredness, joint pain, and depression. This combination of a disappointed, unhappy person, with tiredness, joint pains, and a slightly positive blood test – almost any positive blood test, in fact – is a desperately complex thing to unravel.

'Well…' I say, for the third time, sounding like the policeman in the child's joke, 'the test wasn't *exactly* positive…'

'And it wasn't *exactly* followed up, either…'

True.

Toni/Antonio is now clinging to his mother, bored, pulling and twirling off one of her fingers.

He has a point, the bored child. We *have* been talking for 20 minutes.

'Toni!' she snaps, 'I told you! You need to be quiet when mummy's at the doctor!'

Towards us doctors, Antonio's mum adopts a posture of forgiveness – anyone can make a mistake after all – but she uses our oversight as a weapon from time to time.

Antonio slouches back to those uninteresting toys. Little Toni, now playing the *depressed* cat.

His mother and I have been having this conversation now for 25 minutes.

His mother and I have been having this conversation for *years*.

'Let's focus on the future, eh? How're the rehabilitation exercises?'

Antonio's mother rolls up her eyes – *rehabilitation!* – shifts her weight in the chair, says *'Ooof'*, sighs, changes the subject.

'I have this terrible metallic taste in my mouth…'

Things started to go wrong for Antonio after his audition for Paris. He was 13. I saw him just before he went. His mother was taking him on the train. She was in a rush – all packed and ready to go, but she had run out of her painkillers, and had been told that she needed an appointment to see me. Back when she was the focus of my concern, I always insisted that she make an appointment to see me. I was on a mission to limit, reduce, stop, her many painkillers, which weren't helping, and I thought were holding her back from recovery, and so I would meet her many requests for 'top-up' prescriptions with the request that she see me. It was one of many little battlegrounds with her.

While she went through a shopping list, Antonio stood at her shoulder, an arm protectively around her. He was newly tall, willowy, dressed in tight, fake leopard-skin trousers, a lime green cashmere jumper, and while I negotiated each point on his mother's poisons list, part of my mind, distracted, thought: *Antonio, how do you manage to be whatever it is you are, when nothing in your world enables it? How do you manage to nurture whatever unique identity it is that you have, without even knowing what that identity will be?*

When he came back from Paris, for the first time since early childhood, Antonio had an appointment to see me on his own account. He was limping badly. He had borrowed his mother's stick, which he was using wrongly, but he was clearly in pain. He limped down the corridor, one hand on his mother's arm, the other on the stick. He sat opposite me, silent, confused.

'Antonio's hurt his hip,' his mother says.

The audition had gone well. While Antonio sits in silent discomfort, his mother speaks for him. He had danced before the panel, then performed mime improvisation with a small group of other boys and girls, taken direction, then made a little solo performance which had elicited a patter of applause, which was unusual. Two of the other boys were Russian and spoke no English, but one, Axel, from Munich, spoke some, and they had formed a tentative kind of friendship. Antonio had never spoken before about friends – I had always supposed him to have none.

'And then *this* happens...' she says, indicating her son's left leg, which he holds at an angle to his body, looking at it with curiosity, as if it is no longer his.

'What happened?'

'So *stupid*...' spits his mother.

After a hard day of free movement, dance, choreography and sample lessons, before the evening tour of the residence, perhaps as a kind of indication of reassuring normality to the children and their parents, they had allowed the children out for a picnic tea, and then to run around and play in the ornamental gardens surrounding the conservatoire. The children, initially cautious, but growing in confidence, had lost themselves for an hour, chasing through manicured hedges, around rococo statues, dodging tourists, becoming like puppy dogs.

'They should never have allowed it. It wasn't safe. These are *children*!'

One of them, a confident American girl called Kimmie, had brought a frisbee, and quickly the timid boys had been organised into packs by the girls and they were playing in teams.

'Can you believe it? They were playing frisbee! In a *garden*! In *Paris*!'

And Antonio had leapt to catch a frisbee in flight, had leapt higher and longer than the other child – and I could just picture this, the child with his red hair hanging in the sky in Paris, hanging there for a little longer than was possible for a mortal body – but then he had landed badly.

'How badly?'

His hip had *clicked*.

'So *stupid*!' says his mother, shaking her head. She has dyed her hair I notice. Previously streaked with grey, now lustrous black, thick hair. It made a difference.

'And that's it? His hip just clicked?'

'And he has been in *agony* since then.'

Antonio sits passive and unperturbed, but at this last bit he looks up at me, and nods, says, 'It's really agony!'

Antonio's mother was brought up in a vicarage in Dorset. Despite having been educated for his whole life in Scotland, Antonio's accent has stuck with his mother's. He has these perfect, cut-glass English vowels, which he has used fearlessly in all the playgrounds of all the schools of Craigrothie and Tain. I have no sense of how his father speaks – no recollection of his speech at all – neither its quality nor content.

'Let me look at it.'

I have in my mind a list of possibilities. The ordinary thoughts that a doctor might have, confronting a quite common, modestly difficult technical question: *what is causing Antonio's hip pain? What's the best path to follow to get him walking again?* Because he's hardly walking at all now. He may have limped down the corridor with his mother's stick, but now, in the short distance between the chair and my couch, things seem to have stiffened up, because he can scarcely stand. He huffs and puffs with pain and reaches for his mother's hand, stumbling to the couch. Walking is a huge problem now. Climbing onto the couch, less so. I notice that he flexes his hip to climb up, then abducts it – spreads it wide – to make room. He rests on the couch, says '*Ooof...*' – just like his mother might – and closes his eyes. His mother and I both notice it. She says, 'You're sounding like an old man, Toni!'

There's nothing broken at least, I think. Fracture of the hip is an old person's disease, unless there's bony spread from a cancer, and that's very unlikely indeed in Antonio's case. He might have some kind of rare dancer's stress fracture, made unstable by the bad landing, and I make a mental note to x-ray him and check this out. The pain seems quite inconsistent, varying according to context, and the pain behaviour – the limping, and the 'I'm in pain' noises – are a bit extreme, but that's really quite common, especially with young people. Young people have to learn how to express their pain, just like anyone else.

One of the hard things about assessing pain and injury is to be able reliably to distinguish between behaviours caused by tissue damage – the screaming, for example, of a person trying to walk on the grating ends of broken bones – from those behaviours that are learned and elaborated by a social person to demonstrate to others that they have pain. To understand pain, you have to understand that it has this social, as well as subjective, dimension. It doesn't happen consciously, and there is no clear distinction between *expressing* a pain, and *feeling* it. That is, in the world of pain, if no other, we *are*, or *become*, our actions. Nor is it that one kind of behaviour is more 'genuine' than another – they mix and overlap. Both forms of behaviour are diagnostically important – it makes the difference between giving someone morphine, putting them in a splint and referring them for urgent surgery, or just writing a letter to their sports teacher excusing them from gym. Your decision can change the trajectory of a person's life.

I gently rock his thighs to and fro, and he grasps my hand to make it stop, and I apologise. Rule number one: establish trust. If you hurt a patient without warning, you lose that, and sometimes never get it back. I ask him to flex his thighs, right followed by left, and he manages that, with some effort. When I try to do the same though, gently grasping his ankles and, with warning this time, flexing his hips, gently coaxing them this way and then that, he tenses up. I pause. I say, conversationally, 'So, how do you think the audition went? Do you think you got in?' and Antonio says, as if it were nothing at all, 'Oh yes, they told us, before we left, four of us out of 12 – we got in. Three of the boys, one girl. The others all went home. They're offering to pay for me as well!'

'Wow,' I say, impressed as much by Antonio's insouciance, as by his achievement. 'You must be excited!'

I notice that Antonio is no longer tense. I notice that the range of movement in his hip is now far greater. I keep talking. 'So will you take it? Or are you going to wait and see what London says?'

'Oh, I'll certainly take it! Paris? London? There's no choice!' I laugh, now twisting the hip this way and that, and he seems pain-free, and then Antonio's mum says, 'Tell the doctor if it hurts, Antonio!' and immediately Antonio stiffens up again, which seems significant.

There are countless merely physical causes for Antonio's pain. He might have a slipped cartilage. The soft upper part of his hip bone – the ball part of a ball and socket joint – may have slipped with respect to the bone. He's in the right age group, and it can be precipitated by minimal trauma, but this condition mainly affects overweight and unfit children and Antonio's neither. Also, it's characteristically less painful. But definitely worth mentioning on an x-ray form.

A fibrous cuff surrounds the hip joint – the labrum – and it tears in young, fit people. A labral tear can click, and hurt. A typical performance artist's injury, it would certainly be worth knowing, worth fixing.

A muscle that runs by the inner part of the spine and initiates flexion of the hip joint – the psoas muscle – that clicks too, and can hurt, particularly among athletes. It would be good to diagnose, although the tests I've done for all these are negative.

'I don't know exactly what's going on, Antonio.'

He sits opposite me now. I make eye contact with him, try to create this deliberately exclusive space between us. I want this conversation to take place between him and me. I want his mother somewhere one step outside of that.

'But I don't sense that it is going to be too serious, too big a problem for you. We need to do an x-ray, but I think that it is unlikely to show us very much. It's mainly to exclude some rare things. I think that the thing here is for you to rehabilitate as quickly as possible, to get you back to performing. Let's do the x-ray. I'll see you in a couple of days, and we'll make a concrete plan. How's that sound?'

'Great,' says Antonio, clearly pleased.

'Rehabilitate?' says his mother, clearly sceptical.

———

Was I perpetrating a trick upon Antonio when I examined him? When I distracted him from his symptoms? Then roughly moved his hips around like the hinges on an old wooden deck-chair? I think that his mother thought so; I think that that was, in part, where things started to go wrong. It set up the beginning of a kind of conflict.

Being ill, or having the status of being ill, or being uncertain whether one has, or should adopt that status, is, itself, a harm. Nothing, perhaps, in comparison to the harm caused by, say, a missed fracture, or a missed cancer diagnosis, but a harm none-theless, and a common one. Someone, at some point, has to make a decision, and inevitably decisions are founded in imperfect data.

———

I have in mind another child that I looked after a few years ago. She was 14 as well, when I knew her. Now she will be 24 or 25. I never knew her very well, but I realise now that she changed my outlook on things. My memory of her, for some reason, has sunk down deep, and it lives with me. She *biased* me.

When I knew her, Melanie had been unwell for five years. *Her* illness had started with joint and muscle pain, then pervasive tiredness, insomnia, fluctuating mood, extreme fatigability and slow recovery from exertion, and a progressive inability to participate in school and family life. She had had many tests, from many doctors: of her blood, her hormones, cortisol, nutritional status, trace elements, her guts, intestinal flora, her muscles, including muscle biopsies, her brain, including MRI scans and lumber puncture, her mind, including, reluctantly, psychiatric evaluation: although a person with no knowledge or insight at all, meeting her, would tell in a moment that she wasn't depressed. She seemed psychologically quite resilient, if angry.

When I knew her, she spent most of the time in bed. She propelled herself through her parents' adapted house in a motorised wheelchair. Her mother had given up work to look after her, and the family were in receipt of disability payments. She was bright; she radiated a sense of competence and *coping*. She was on very high doses of opiates for unexplained muscle and joint pain, and that was the reason for my visits. The doctors principally involved in caring for her were frightened; they visited regularly in order to keep some kind of control over her consumption, although she seemed to me to be as different as it is possible to be from a typical opiate-seeking addict.

'They think I'm turning into a junkie!' she said lightheartedly as she propelled herself into the room where she kept her meds, laid out in careful order on a table, with a schedule and a diary, to be helpful to me, which it was, hugely. Her mother was proud of her maturity and her stoicism.

The thing was, she had been given no clear diagnosis, at any time. She didn't even have an *unclear* diagnosis. She had some labels which stuck for a while, and then came off again, but these seemed to be no more than descriptions for gatherings of symptoms, some of which may have been helpful, and others not. A label isn't the same as a diagnosis.

I am haunted by her memory because she was so young. Because she was very clever and capable, and because I liked her. There seemed to me, in her case, to be so much at stake. There seemed to be a *lifetime* at stake. Yet there was no plan. No *end game*. There was no one in charge, and there seemed nowhere else to go, other than to escalate her dosage of opiates until what? There seemed no one in charge of her case, and even if there had been, even if I were to *make myself that person,* which was presumptuous, as she certainly didn't accord me that, or any, status, there seemed nowhere even to begin a conversation about how to recover. What would be the first step in Melanie's case to begin to recover?

In Melanie's case, there must have been a first doctor. A first casting off into choppy water, the start of a voyage which had led her to where she was, when I met her. There must have been a day when things got started. I looked in her records. I was curious, I wanted to understand. It was back in a time when records could be very brief indeed. All they said in her case was: 'Muscle pains. Child feels TATT (*tired all the time*). Not attending school, wants letter.' There wasn't anything more dramatic, or interesting than that. That appeared to be how it all started. If that doctor, wide awake and vigilant, his hand on the tiller, the other on the main-sheet, had set a different line of sail, perhaps just a few degrees into the wind, might the outcome have been changed? Might some harm have been avoided?

It is possible that I have over-generalised from the case of Melanie – from how I recall and interpret it. I have, perhaps, allowed the memory of her case to affect me too much. I have moved on now, to a different city in a different country, and I have lost track of her. I can't check now. I can't ask her. I don't know what became of her.

I think that that first doctor is in the same position as the doctor facing the questions *Might this be a fracture? Or cancer? A destructive bacterial infection? Or the first presentation of an arthritis destined to permanently cripple?* Although Melanie has no such physically destructive process, the jeopardy is the same. In Melanie's case, the outcome seemed just as disabling, just as life-altering. A diagnosis of cancer, or arthritis, or a fracture, can be the work of minutes, provided the penny drops. The diagnostic challenge in Melanie's case is more complex. We have no easy words or labels or categories to describe meaningfully what it is that ailed Melanie. On that first day when she walked into a doctor's office, announcing that she was ill, we have no words to describe what it is that we feared for her.

I would like not to be that first doctor, who wrote 'TATT' (*tired all the time*). Note for school.' And failed to see the gathering clouds, the dark waters that she was sailing into.

———

When Antonio comes back to see me, a few days later, I think *oh, hell*.

'So much for rehabilitation,' says his mother, with a stoical, forgiving smile.

He is back on the stick – his own this time, and someone has taught him to use it. He hops along with something like agility beside his mother, who strides now quite boldly beside him. The father stays in the waiting room, guarding coats and bags while mother and child do the business. They sit. Antonio's mother hands me an envelope, 'GP' written on it in pointy accusing letters. I think *oh, hell…*

'He just couldn't take the pain any more. He had to be rushed into hospital in the middle of the night. They had to give him *morphine* for the pain.'

'Gosh,' I say.

'He had *bloods* done. And a scan. They thought he might have an infection in the joint, or even a fracture.' The accusation isn't far off. I can feel it coming. 'One of the doctors even said that it could be cancer.'

I skim read the letter, trying to gather information, listen to Antonio's mother, contain my own worry, disaster-manage, all at the same time.

'I'm glad that the bloods … and the x-ray … and the scan are all normal…' I say, a little tentatively, trying to de-escalate. 'What did they say it was in the end?'

'They gave us these. They told us to get more from you.'

She hands me a couple of strips of painkillers. Tramadol. Very commonly prescribed. Appeared in the 1990s as an option for severe post-operative pain, they are said to be a little safer than conventional opiates, and cause fewer side effects, such as vomiting and constipation. Now they are prescribed for pretty much everything: it's not so uncommon for people to take them for a simple headache.

I see in my memory a ghost image of a child in a wheelchair, propelling herself from room to room telling me, chirpily, about her dosage schedule for her pain. I want to say to Antonio '*Don't take these! Don't take these!*' But I can't find the words to say even that.

'What did they tell you the problem was?'

'They said that Toni needed an urgent orthopaedic review. They said that you had to organise that, but that it should be urgent. They thought he probably needed another body scan to make the diagnosis.'

'Did *anyone* tell you what they thought the problem might be?'

I tried as hard as I could. I showed Antonio that he could walk well without his crutch. With a little support, he walked normally down the corridor and back; with encouragement, he went without the supporting hand on his elbow, and he walked, it seemed to me, without pain. I avoided the toxic 'rehabilitation' word. But when I suggested to him that he do more of this at home – the more the better in fact – his mother said, 'After we've seen the specialist though, obviously…' and I hadn't the authority left in me to argue the point, and said, 'Obviously.'

And I warned him, warned him hard, against the powerful painkillers that I was signing for, how they would affect him, how they would rob him of his agility and his sharpness, depress his mood, slow his body, knowing, knowing all the time, that the signing of this poisonous prescription would be a gesture far stronger than the force of any cautious words, and yet still I signed it.

———

Every day I see people with disorders and illnesses that have profound physical effects, but nothing to see that is broken. Nothing to measure or detect.

People who have pain, who limp, who are constantly and unfathomably tired. People disabled by headaches or backaches, abdominal bloating, or diarrhoea, or constipation, or gas, or peeing glass, or peeing all the time. Weaknesses, in any part, that come or go, or are here to stay. Fits and funny turns, or thrashing around for no reason. Rashes and funny feelings or funny tastes, or some alteration in any part of the body that is so strange that it can't be described with words. People burdened by perceptions that indicate to them that they are *really* ill. Symptoms which *could* represent something terribly serious: something incapacitating, life-altering, the beginning of the end, but which, in these patients at least, don't. At least not in the sense that they fear.

These sorts of disorders, this pool of symptoms, which evade easy physical attribution, have always been with us. They have always troubled patients and their doctors. Nowadays, perhaps more preoccupied than we once were with *feelings,* we tend to think that there is something primarily mental about them. Something consequential upon how people think, which then somehow affects their physical functioning. We haven't always thought about it like that. To think about things in that way, you need certain tools and ideas. You need, in the first place, the idea that there is a mind, and that there is a body, and that they consist of different substances. You need to think that these two substances somehow interact with one another to create the universe that we experience, and you need ideas and theories about how that might happen. The idea that this might present a problem of metaphysics is an idea as old as philosophy itself. The idea that that might make you ill is much more recent. Perhaps it is our ability to think and talk in this way that makes it possible for us to suffer from these kinds of illnesses. The gap between the mind and the body is a mysterious and baffling place: full of obscure language, paradoxes and tricks, and utterly devoid of solace for a person in pain, who fears that the person treating him thinks his suffering *imaginary*.

There is something mental about *all* disorders, of course. Ask any sick person how they feel; they will tell you. There is definitely something mental about how it feels to have disseminated cancer, or multiple sclerosis, or a gunshot wound. This kind of interaction, where the connection runs from the physical to the mental, seems unproblematic and intuitive. It can work the other way as well: there are kinds of mental phenomena which seem to have straightforward, catastrophic physical consequences: such as liking to smoke, resulting in lung cancer, or liking to drink alcohol, resulting in liver failure. Driving too fast. The buzz of solo rock climbing. Or a purely mental phenomenon such as despair, leading to the physical consequences of self-injury or suicide. Chronic insomnia, and its associations with dementia, depression, premature coronary vascular disease, early death. But these are not the kind of mind/body phenomena that fret us, at least philosophically.

The kinds of illnesses I am concerned with are different. In these disorders, the connection between the primary mental phenomenon (whatever it is) and its physical, perceptual, symptomatic consequences, seems *necessarily* obscure. It is as if there is something about the obscurity of the connection that makes these conditions what they are. Perhaps it is only that strange conceptual space in which they flourish that has the necessary conditions for their propagation. If we didn't carry these complex embodied minds, we wouldn't suffer from these complex illnesses.

Whatever the nature of these conditions, they are very hard to talk about. Especially with a sufferer. To be told when you feel unwell that your disorder is somehow caused by 'how you think' is implausible. It seems so palpably untrue that pain can arise from your mind, it has the effect of denying the reality of your experience. This is extraordinarily offensive. It translates as 'not real', 'imagined', 'made up', 'all in your head'. It seems to make a liar of the sufferer. No matter what the words you choose, or your skill in saying them, that's what you seem to be saying.

———

I played a small part in the wrecking of little Antonio's life. It shames me.

What I didn't anticipate, what I hadn't seen, in my enthusiasm for Antonio's *specialness*, was how vulnerable he was. How vulnerable was the garden of his mind to being overrun by weeds. As a painkiller, the tramadol worked fine in its blunt and facile way, at least for a bit. The pain got better, but in every other way, the boy was harmed.

He didn't perform for the several weeks it took to establish that he would wait three months to see a specialist on the NHS. It seemed to his mother too dangerous for the boy to leap, twist, mime, dance, lest whatever had been wrong be made worse, and so he didn't for months. They paid for a private scan in the end, which was normal. By the time he was followed up in the NHS clinic and his illness left unexplained, the injury was a memory. Paris was a memory. The leaping for the frisbee, the American girl, Kimmie, who had encouraged the boys to race and trip and leap like little dogs around the ornamental gardens of the ballet school, were all memories. It seemed to take so little to change the trajectory of that boy's life. Just one step: an ill-considered leap into the air. His hip *clicked* when he landed.

It was bad for Antonio not to perform. His body, changing anyway, changed badly. He lost muscle, stopped eating, fearing fat, became plump anyway, lost his child confidence. His skin no longer glowed, was speckled now with acne, and his girlish red hair became oily and lank. Puberty, of course. Perhaps the Antonio *I* had admired was just the immature form, the skittish kid, the gamboling juvenile; perhaps something was set in Antonio that all along he was destined to thicken with age, that what was emerging now was the *echt* Antonio, the real one, but I doubt it. I still see myself as an agent of the harm.

'You need to get moving again, Antonio. Get back to the theatre.'

The walking stick is a fixture now, as is the changed gait – there's a bit of a waddle as he walks, his hip stabilisers weakened from immobility and the weight that he has put on. Athletes' bodies go to mush when they stop. He slumps in the chair and scowls.

His mother has started going to the gym. She has slimmed down, stays on her feet, does all the talking. She is energised and more alive than I have ever seen her. She declaims from a list, expressing each point and detail of her son's illness with a raised forefinger. It's hard for me to get a word in. Things have moved on for Antonio. His health concerns read like a schedule of building works.

The private orthopaedic surgeon has suggested that he see a rheumatologist to 'rule out' juvenile arthritis, and the rheumatologist has suggested that he have some 'baseline bloods' done. As his mother talks, I try to look up information on the computer to ascertain which of these bloods he may already have had. 'The hip pain is better on the tramadol, though *obviously* we still need to get to the bottom of it, but another doctor meanwhile has started a different drug, called amitriptyline, an antidepressant, which can cause tiredness, blurred vision, urinary retention and constipation as side-effects but they still think that that is worth soldiering on with and can we increase the dose? But the main problem today is a rash, but before you tell us that it's just a side effect from the tramadol, it's not, because Toni,' (who stares at his shoes, which once were fake lizard skin and now are plastic trainers) 'has been up all night itching, haven't you? So can we see a dermatologist or an allergy specialist to rule out a skin issue too?'

'You *just* need to get going again!'

My frustration is coming through – even I can hear it. That 'just' word must feel like an assault to Antonio, but I battle on anyway. 'You *just* need to stop the painkillers, stop all the drugs. You *just* need to get back to your dancing and your mime!'

'But what about the pain? Whenever he stops the tramadol, the pain comes straight back.'

'Paracetamol? Ibuprofen?' I suggest, already knowing the answer, which comes back to me like a ping-pong ball.

'We tried them months ago. They made him sick and didn't help.'

Antonio looks at the floor. I look at Antonio's head. His mother looms down on me, face framed in a mass of black, angry hair. An angry triangle. Even the *scent* she wears seems angry.

'It's not right for the boy to be like this. He just sits in his room, even when he's *not* in pain. If it's not his skin, it's his bladder – it hurts to pee, doesn't it, Toni? – and if it's not his bladder, it's his stomach. We're up all night too, because he's scratching and itching, moaning and complaining. I don't see how *stopping* the pain killers is going to help, when he's in so much pain!'

Bladder, hip, skin, gut, soul: every time I whack one symptom, another pops up.

I think: I might as well be saying *'just stop being ill!'*

'You might as well be saying *just stop being ill!'* says Antonio's mother.

Change tack.

'How's your mood been, Antonio?'

'Bloody awful, what do you expect?' snaps his mother. 'He's lost everything. Everything!'

'What do *you* think, Antonio? How's your mood been?'

'Okay.' Says Antonio.

'Okay…' I say, stuck, bashing on.

'You see, sometimes when people have physical symptoms, it can be helpful to find out a little about whether there is anything that might be making them unhappy … that might be contributing to their symptoms. Sometimes it can be helpful to see a psychologist, or a specialist like that, to see if *they* can help…'

The ice beneath my feet … cracks … and creaks…

'... so rather than just refer on to another specialist about your *skin*, or your *bladder*, I was thinking that we might get a psychologist...'

The ice beneath my feet ... creaks ... and cracks...

'... to assess you, to see if there are any underlying *emotional* factors that...'
    ... CRACKS.

'Are you saying that this is *all in my head*?'

Antonio looks up at me, for the first time, in a long time, and I can see that his face is streaked with tears. He has been weeping all this time, and I haven't seen it. His mother looks horrified.
    'No! I'm not saying that it's *all in your head*, I'm saying...'
    'Then what are you saying?'

———————

I guess I *am* saying that it's all in Antonio's head.

That delicate, finely tuned instrument – the accidental creation that he was – plays out of tune now. The bits are all there, arranged just as they always were – the scans show us that – but all the music is gone, the harmony lost. I can see it in his eyes. This bewildered sense of loss. A baffled look.

I asked the advice of a colleague, Dr Marks, a consultant in my local district general, who makes a speciality of managing hard cases: very sick people with normal bodies. She's a diagnostician, a doctor with an open mind. Some areas still have one or two, slaving away under the radar in the NHS, although they are becoming rare. She invited me to join her in clinic one morning – to be a medical student again.

We see a series of sick people, all ordinary, all extraordinary, in their own way.

One twisted something in his back a year or two ago, hoisting a bag of coal. Although litigation with his employer has made him rich, enough to buy his flat at least, his back won't straighten now. He walks, twisted hard to the left, and the muscle spasm has spread to affect his arms and his legs. He played competitive football before his injury – he'd like to get back to it. Since his case was settled, his symptoms have worsened. He is abject. His gait, his manner of walking, has something of the theatre about it – he moves like the back end of a pantomime horse. His face is dark with pain. He's not making it up.

Some are angry. Some hate their doctors, some hate their ex-wives, some are fantastically well-informed, advocates for their illness, some are depressed, or anxious – but most aren't. Most are ordinary, in their own way.

One has been mislabeled and has a rare neurological condition that can be mitigated by stopping the medications that are provoking it – this is rare.

Most are stuck, making the best they can of their situation, struggling on through life – education, work, parenthood, old age – for as long as they can, until they can't struggle any longer. Few, if any, are cured. People just seem to manage. Individual symptoms recede, new ones take their place.

Dr Marks says, 'I prefer to talk about "functional symptoms". "Psychosomatic" is used as a derogatory expression in the media, like "hypochondriac" and that's now how people understand these terms – as coded insults. "Psychogenic" is too psychological. It doesn't capture the physical reality of illness, its tangibility, and so people understand that as "imagining it". "Somatising" is too unfamiliar, "conversion disorder" too technical sounding, too Freudian, and "hysterical" is just medieval: cruel and misleading.

'"Medically unexplained symptoms" was popular for a while, but is useless as a therapeutic label. People hear it as an admission of ignorance or incompetence, which I guess in some ways it is. "Abnormal illness behaviour" is a way of blaming the victim.

'I like to use the metaphor of a computer with a software malfunction. So, the computer is physically normal, but the programme it runs isn't working. For those patients who aren't familiar with computers, I talk about a piano or a guitar that is out of tune. The word "functional" captures that nicely, I think.'

Dr Marks spends an hour with each new patient. She fought for that privilege, to have the time to care properly for her difficult patients, and this dispensation of time is always under threat. She meticulously lists each symptom until there are no new symptoms to list, and her patients, sensing her thoroughness, awaken: they sit up, focus, give her their best account. She explores each symptom with questions and deft examinations, bright lights shone into eyes, tuning forks, coloured pins, tendon hammers, until she has run each item of suffering down to a plausible explanation. She explains which of the symptoms are physical, and which 'functional', and explains what she means by that. She uses her computer analogy repeatedly: explains it again, and once again. Her patients listen to her, intently. They don't seem to interrupt her in the way that they would interrupt me. Her meticulous history-taking and examination – her *performance* of competence – have earned her their attention and respect. She has built the foundations for authority. She tests again their understanding of her explanation, and asks whether they believe her.

'Everything depends on understanding. If a person doesn't understand, or doesn't believe you, then they can't possibly get better. That's in the nature of functional illness.'

It is as if, making their own way through the woods, each of these people, once as strong or fragile as you or me, has taken an unmarked turning and become lost, taken a path into sickness.

If this were a journal of psychotherapy, I would provide an interpretative map with landmarks marked and a compass, or a guide with a cloak and staff to walk with them a while, to help them find their own route through.

Of Antonio, I might say that it was *his mother* that was to blame all along. *Harsh but true,* I might pronounce. (It always seems to be the mother that gets the blame, although Antonio's is more loving, more attentive, than most.) I might say that it was she that infected her son with her disappointment. I might say that, vampire-like, she sucked the vitality from her son. I might say that her son learned everything he needed to know about the performance of illness from his mother: it was *expected* of him. I might say: free himself of his mother and he will be free of what ails him. It's *her* fault.

Or, conversely, I might say that the fault was *his*: not his mum at all. I might say that, faced with the reality, the implications of his talent, the fear of adulthood and leaving home, illness was a safer place for him to be. That the boy just wasn't ready to leave the nest.

Or it might be that, mediated by my skill as a psychotherapist, Antonio might have disclosed to me that thing he had feared to tell anyone. Perhaps the other boys at the conservatoire were being sexually touched by a dance master. Perhaps he was afraid of Paris.

Or that he, Antonio, during that visit to Paris, had felt in himself the first stirrings of a homosexual longing for Axel from Munich, and the spectre of love so disturbed him that he took refuge in illness to flee it.

All or none of these contradictory explanations might be true. They might *feel* true, to Antonio, or to me. Compellingly so, perhaps. But to know whether any were would be impossible. They're just stories, after all, some helpful, some less so. Who could tell whether any contains any truth at all? In any case, I tried. I did refer Antonio to see a child and adolescent psychologist in the teeth of his and his mother's objection. It was a referral made so unskilfully, and so unlikely to be met with success, that it makes me grieve to recollect it. He attended one appointment then didn't go back, so we will never know whether that would have worked, whether a psychological interpretation, valid or not, might have proved helpful to him.

I didn't see Antonio for a while.

The hip pain was gradually forgotten, but was subsumed in chronic low-level bladder pain. However hard he tried, he just couldn't seem to empty his bladder. We blamed the drug, amitriptyline – it says prominently on the list of side effects 'urinary retention' – but stopping the drug made no difference.

Precipitated by his now desperate mother, he had repeated attendances at accident and emergency departments. He was seen by a variety of junior doctors. Tired and overworked, one suggested the possibility of 'nerve damage' from the drugs. That didn't help much, but the idea certainly stuck. Another, I think in desperation, passed a catheter to finally prove that his bladder was empty, and that seemed to help a lot: Antonio got back to school for a bit, everything seemed better, but then it recurred. Another doctor ordered an MRI scan of his abdomen. It showed some minor damage to the kidneys: some widening of the ureter, which passes from the kidney to the bladder, a problem from childhood, previously undetected. Seemed like an answer, at last, for a while, but it wasn't.

An MRI of the brain ruled out MS or a spinal cord injury, and a urology nurse specialist taught Antonio the technique of intermittent self-catheterisation so that, once or twice a week, if things got really bad, Antonio could empty his bladder *himself*. It helped, enormously: most days the boy passed a catheter, relieved himself of a teaspoonful or two of retained urine, but the amounts became less and less, and the pain started to grow more.

A urologist organised some urodynamic studies. Antonio sat in a room with leaky old men and drank bottles of water and peed into a bucket while a nurse scanned his bladder. The tests were normal, and the letters between the doctors, copied to *GP*, me, took on a slightly snide tone. Where was all this water going, if he wasn't peeing, eh? Doctors chortled behind his back, rolled their eyes in frustration, straightened their faces when his mother came into the room. No one said anything to Antonio or his mother. No one was brave enough to express the accusation: that someone somewhere wasn't telling the truth. The suspicion caught on – never explicit, but coded – that Antonio's illness was *factitious,* that is, he was making it up, faking it, deceiving people, his mother, his doctors, himself. Once thought, the suspicion couldn't be un-thought.

Sensing skepticism, Antonio's mother started to take photos on her smartphone of Antonio trying to squeeze out drops of urine. He would press on his bladder, he would sit, he would stand, he would writhe, he would run the taps, then squeeze out another drop or two, weep salty tears. Between times, Antonio started dribbling. Try as he might, he couldn't stay dry. Needing access to a toilet at all times, he started skipping school completely.

Antonio developed chronic urinary retention with overflow. His scans were normal, his bladder too. But unable to wee, he was seen by a urologist, who passed a permanent catheter. He couldn't *not* wee, he already had scars on the kidney: he would have developed kidney failure. He needed that catheter. Imagine that: being a 16-year-old boy with a urinary catheter.

Antonio's mother left his father. Perhaps it was the pressure of having a child with complex, chronic ill health. One day the father wasn't there anymore. It seemed to make little difference to Antonio. As often happens when an unhappy marriage ends, his mother seemed, somehow, unburdened by the separation. She no longer needed a stick to walk. She started wearing make-up, changed her hair, practised Tai-Chi, changed her posture, the whole way her body moved.

Antonio was flabby-thin, pale, ghostly. Walking became a problem, not so much because of bladder pain, but because he was weak. He hardly ate: how could he, with his pain? And he didn't need to anyway. Scarcely moving, he had no energy to expend. He stopped attending doctors because none took him seriously, none listened to him; they were a waste of time. He hardly left the house. He seemed to spend his life on Facebook, checking the internet for the symptoms of bladder stones and schistosomiasis, reading fan fiction, standing at the toilet, fussing with his catheter, staring at his bedroom ceiling.

———

'You said it!' says Antonio, pinning me with his violet blue eyes. 'These were your exact words!'

'But!'

'You said, "it's all in your head!"'

'But … but… I'm sorry, that wasn't what I meant…'

'But it's what you said…'

———

A case conference has been called. All the people involved in Antonio's care, all to meet in one room. We should have done that a long time ago. It seems so obvious, in hindsight, with all that harm, already done. We should have met months ago. Years ago. Once everyone was in the same room, sitting around a table, it seemed to take just moments to find clarity.

His urology nurse told us what we knew already: that the scans and urodynamic studies were all normal. Nothing we were doing was helping. Her guess was that he could pee just fine, but was now too embarrassed to say. 'He needs a way out from all this. He needs to climb down. He needs to find some route to get better.'

His neurologist said, 'It's not his wiring…'

An interventional radiologist, called in with a view to passing the tiniest imaginable tube to bypass his bladder altogether, said, surprised: 'So you mean he's not even got a urinary problem?'

The psychiatrist, who was taking notes said: 'He seemed keen to convince me that he wasn't crazy. I was pretty convinced that he wasn't crazy.'

Someone, not me, said, 'It's all functional really, isn't it? It's all just functional.'

Just functional. What does that mean?

'So who's going to tell *him* that?'

All eyes on me; I said nothing.

'I'm sorry Antonio.' I let the apology sit a while. The other doctors looked embarrassed for me. I *feel* embarrassed.

'I'm sorry. I shouldn't have said anything that would have led you to believe that.' I let that one sit, too.

Then Antonio says, 'I used to trust you. You listened. You really seemed to care. You seemed interested in the theatre and the mime and so on. Then you told me that it was all in my head, and then you just seemed to stop listening.'

His mother says, 'We all felt that way. We trusted you. We felt really let down.'

'I'm sorry.'

An apology to work as an apology has to be unqualified. The inevitable 'but' always spoils it. I work hard to resist the 'but'. I clamp my jaws down upon its slippery tail and won't let it wriggle free. No 'buts' today.

'I'm sorry that I told you that it was all in your head.' I swallow hard. No 'buts'.

The other doctors look at their feet.

'So what do you *really* think is wrong?'

'I think you have a functional disorder.'

Antonio cocks his head to one side. His mother raises her eyebrows. The others look up from their feet.

'It means that … it means … it's as if you were a computer. It's as if all the electronics were working, and the hard drive's fine, it's not got wet or been dropped or broken the screen, but…'

'… but the software's not working? One of the nurses told me that once, one night in A&E. That seemed to make a lot of sense at the time. Then another doctor came in and told me that I needed a catheter change…'

'… It's like a computer virus. Everything working mechanically, but it still doesn't function.'

'That's how I feel. As if everything's jammed. It's all out of sync. What should I do?'

———

I have this very strong subjective sense of a central, essential self, who sits in the cockpit of a body: an agent, that controls his world; a subject, perceiving things about his world. I think it's likely that everyone I know experiences the world in that way – I think that it forms the fundamental grammar of experience. Maybe that's the source of the problem. Maybe this grammar of subjectivity misleads.

I think that in the moment of an action, we *are* our action. In the moment of intending, we are our intention. When we perceive, we *are* our perception: in a moment of pain, we *are* our pain. Our identity consists of these passing moments of action and awareness, strung like beads upon a thread of memory. Our compelling sense of that stable, unchanging subjective 'I' is an artefact of memory.

Dr Marks's cure seemed to consist mainly in undoing harms.

Imagine this. You were never very resilient in the first place. You might have thought you were, but then you became ill, and that has robbed you of the resilience that you once had. The opiates that you have been prescribed make you tired. They diminish your motivation. They depress your mood. In the long term, they *lower* your threshold to pain. They make you more indifferent to your suffering. They have changed who you are. The new doctor says they need to be stopped. But each reduction in dose brings a flare of demoralising pain. Similarly, the sedatives and anti-convulsants you have been prescribed wrap you in a warm cloak of indifference. They make you *feel* better. But the new doctor says that if you are ever to truly recover, they will have to be stopped. But as they are withdrawn, the world seems once again a cold, loveless place. The dose is progressively reduced, and there is a painful sharpening of awareness and perception – an anguish in the world that you had almost forgotten existed.

The doctor says you have *learned* to be ill – that the lesson needs to be unlearned. The unlearning is gruelling, and needs to be practised. You feel like a child again, unwillingly put to homework. Repeated, pointless practice of *being well*, hour after hour.

The bent man will endure months of exercise and physiotherapy to be straight again. If he neglects the discipline for a day, the spasms will return.

The tottering person on her stick will need to learn to walk again without it, retraining softened muscles, relearning to balance, and she will be full of fear, and sometimes she will fall.

To recover from a functional illness, you need to do the opposite of everything that your illness is prompting you to do. The weary person you have become, floored with pain, has to become active and engage in exercise. You might never have taken exercise in your life before, and know no one who has. I knew a woman once who was 20 kilos overweight and suffered pain.

When she tried to run, she waddled and wobbled and she said to me that young men would slow their cars, open windows, toot their horns and shout at her 'Miss Piggy!' But to recover from functional illness, you *need* to re-enter the world and it may feel like the world doesn't want you. The world looks down on the functionally ill.

Your new doctor has told you that you need to get back to work, but there is no work for you. You are out-competed by people who are fitter and stronger, better educated and better looking. The prospect of job hunting both humiliates and terrifies. Your new doctor talks about you coming off benefits. He doesn't seem to understand that that means you will have no money.

To recover from a functional illness you need to alter what you *do*, what you *feel*, what you *think*. You have to do everything that feels most difficult. You have to change what you *are*, or what your illness has made you become.

I think there could scarcely be anything harder.

I see Antonio every two weeks or so. Antonio is 17 now, and he comes to see me on his own. My cure for him consists of undoing harm. My cure for him consists of not doing very much at all. The metaphor of 'function' works well: it makes sense to him. We no longer fret about what is in his head and what is in his body, what is real, and what isn't, and what these concepts even mean. The hostility has gone from our relationship. We focus on what he's doing, what he's thinking, how well he's functioning. I give a little homework, which he hardly ever does, and I monitor his progress. We agree that any medicine that isn't clearly helping we should stop. We stop all of his medication.

I find that if I don't ask him about his symptoms, he doesn't raise them. We don't talk about his bladder anymore, nor his hip, nor his skin, his bowels nor any part of his body.

I know he has stopped using the catheters because he stopped ordering them. We never speak of it. Sometimes when he sits, he clasps his lower stomach; sometimes he looks a little stiff in the hip when he stands from sitting, catches himself saying 'Ooof!' but he just laughs and shrugs his shoulders. He attends school most days now, building up from a faltering start. He's missed most of the crucial years, all his important exams, and so will have to take the long way round, through college, if he is to progress in his education.

He has started walking his dog. His father bought him a dog, to his mother's disgust, and he takes it on the beach most evenings. He is still flabby-thin, but he has started jogging a little: he doesn't want his dog to get arthritis or diabetes. We never talk about mime or theatre. He seems almost to have forgotten that he ever danced. He now stays weekdays and alternate weekends with his father on a pull-out couch in the sitting room. His dad helps him with his homework.

Antonio was an unusual child. He is an unusual young man. It emerges that we share a passion for classical music. He had always loved it, he and his father, all those years, but in our many conversations the subject had never come up. Why would it?

This morning I am running late. I am always running late. This is bad: I've been chin-wagging with Antonio again, who wanted me to know that he has been listening to Wagner. He's just discovered Wagner.

'… I was listening to *Tristan*? You know it? The opera? There's a chord right at the beginning, it's like it defines the whole of the rest of the piece. It comes from this dark silence – from nowhere – but it fills the whole space of the music, unresolved, uncertain, like it could take you anywhere! And it goes on like that, on and on, totally unresolved, filled with uncertainty, for hours, right to the end! It's brilliant! It's like you hear that chord for the first time and you think you've just got to go and rethink your whole life! *Your whole life!*'

Antonio the *Enthusiastic*.

I'm thinking *is this even medicine?*

I'm thinking that the hero of this story will be Antonio.

Shangalang

Roxi's okay, really.

I said goodbye to her, I suspect for the last time. I told her I thought she would be okay. I had stood up long before she was anywhere near finished what she was trying to say. There's no natural end to Roxi's discourse, and no interrupting – never any interrupting. She senses it, with an exquisite, hair-trigger resentment. She has no problem expressing resentment. So, as always, I am standing by my open door, making the broad farewell gesture with my left arm so that she might get the hint – *it's time to go now!* – and she does, at last. She stands, and talking all the while, clutching her prescription to her breast, she makes to leave. And then, hostage to some instinct for kindness, I place a hand on her shoulder. It is intended to be conciliatory and reassuring, the lightest of touches. I'm not usually a 'touchy' kind of person. I'm quite formal, like to keep my distance, but over the years Roxi and I have journeyed a long way together. I say, a little choked, 'You're okay, Roxi. You'll be okay…'

Perhaps I was expecting something in return. Like 'Aye, you're okay too, Doctor,' or even, 'Thanks for everything, Doctor. You've really helped … you've always been there for me…', but no, not today. Not ever. It's a ridiculous thought. There's nothing worse than a needy doctor. Doctors who confuse their own emotional needs with those of their patients. They're the worst.

She shakes my hand off her shoulder, a little roughly, scowls, says, 'Aye, sure, that'll be right,' but in sarcastic mode. Roxi knows well what lies ahead. She's been there before. She's not okay at all. Roxi's going to be sent to prison. She's sure to be. The world's shit-scared of the likes of Roxi.

She's about my age – mid to late fifties. We've lived the same decades pretty much, she and I, we have that in common. She is tiny in frame, with dyed, thinning honey blonde hair with the beginnings of grey in the roots; she's dressed all in black today, a sheer little black suit with a skirt, plunging low decolletage and traces of maroon lace peeking through. She has been to court the previous day, at least so I gather from what I understand of what she tells me, so I'm getting the last of her best wardrobe. There is sweat, smoke and a glassy, sharp scent to cover it all. It's the smell of late night bars, the end of the party, one last song on the juke-box, and she's down to her last cigarette. It's how I imagine the smell of women's prison.

She's done a really bad thing, and she's going down for it.

———

She missed her last appointment, which isn't like her at all, then left a message to say that she'd been in the cells, so I fitted her in specially so that she doesn't run out of methadone. If Roxi runs out of methadone, there will be hell to pay – by me, by Roxi, by society as a whole – and I will go a long-ish way to prevent that from happening. But at the same time, I won't just leave her a prescription for a week, or a month, or longer. I insist on seeing her. No carte blanche for Roxi.

With patients on a prescription for methadone, I seem to have chanced upon a policy which makes life just a little bit difficult – for them, and for me. For each person I deal with, I build into that individual relationship just the right level of difficulty. A little wall or barrier that you have to step over in order to get the goods. So there are certain things that I insist on. You have to turn up on time. You have to treat me with some respect. You have to turn up in person, and you mustn't be 'gouching' (actively intoxicated with drugs) or drunk. You mustn't be armed, and you mustn't be carrying drugs or injecting or burning equipment. You have to pick up your prescription yourself, in person, and you mustn't swear at me directly, at least not too much, and never ever threaten. You mustn't chuck urine specimens at me, or threaten to do so, and the urine that you submit for drugs testing has to be yours, and no one else's. These aren't rules which I have consciously invented – more situations which have cropped up with sufficient regularity for me to have had to adopt rules to govern them. In exchange for observing my rules, I will treat you with respect. I shall try to learn to like you, and help you as much as I can, with the very limited means at my disposal, and within the constraints imposed by my own personal limitations of tolerance, patience, kindness and knowledge, to make whatever it is that you wish to make of the life that you have been given – which is, for starters, in every single case, in my experience, without exception, to not be addicted to heroin any more.

So I make life just a little bit difficult. I put in your way little barriers that must be stepped over to earn the respect that I already owe you and the care that I'm paid to provide you. I'm aware of how patronising that seems. How paternalistic. I didn't set out with these rules in mind. They have simply evolved. Have a pee sample chucked at you a couple of times, then you can judge me.

I think that it is the process – of setting tiny, realisable challenges, and rewarding the successful confrontation of these challenges with respect (and methadone) – that is the treatment. The rest – the checking of blood-borne viruses, the titrating of doses and changing to other substitute prescriptions, and the writing of letters to lawyers, social workers and housing officers, the treating of terrible abscesses in arms and groins and legs and penises and everywhere, the constant battle to reduce and simplify the prescriptions for toxic and unnecessary drugs that this population of people end up being given – is all peripheral. What matters is the relationship. The setting of little challenges. The demanding of a certain level of respect. The rewarding of respect with respect, medical care, a little kindness and methadone.

But Roxi really has done a bad thing.

She looks terrible today. Usually she fizzes: volatile with passion, energy, rage or chemicals. Usually, she is talking at me from the get-go, from the moment that she stands up in the waiting room, about her dog's lustrous hair and how bad Coco smells, or the iniquities of the criminal justice system, or about a bright blue light she witnessed, shining over Craigentinny late one Saturday night, or about a prison officer who called her 'Jelly-Baby' when she was visiting her ex-husband, Jelly-Boy, in gaol. Roxi's conversation has a fragmented, hard-to-capture, hallucinatory quality. But today she is subdued. She still has bed hair, and she has a black eye. She has slept in her clothes. She is a little shaky. She sits down, head bowed and I think *please don't cry*, which is fatal because she immediately starts to cry.

I say nothing. I just wait. She sobs. I bring her a paper towel and she blows her nose, wipes her eyes, hands the towel back to me, and I take it between thumb and forefinger and bin it.

'I'd've expected it from anyone. Anyone [*sob*]. Anyone other than Jelly-Boy. [*Sob*] [*Pause*]'

'What?'

'They've took everything. They stole my phone.' But she *has* her phone, right there in front of her, sitting on my desk in its rhinestone Snapple. Battered, worse for wear, but definitely there: it's *her* phone.

'They got my cards and my tablet. They went through my bag and took everything. All my money, my keys, they've even cut off my electricity!' She snaps her finger, unsuccessfully, tries again, gives up. 'I bet you didnae even know they could do that. Just like that. Nae electricity. You'd have thought it of anyone sooner than Jelly-Boy.'

'But I thought that Jelly-Boy was in prison...'

Jelly-Boy is being detained for life in a state hospital – on a technicality, according to Roxi. He cut a man's throat in a pub toilet ear to ear, she once told me, making a finger-across-throat gesture. Ear to ear, with a defiant gleam in her eye. '... but Jelly-Boy was never like that with me. Niver! With me he's the gentlest man in the world, soft as a butterfly, sweet as a flower, and I'm the only girl that has ever understood him.'

She takes out a crumpled lace hanky and dabs at the tears in her smudged black eyes. 'Oh aye, *he's* in prison. It was his *friends*. They came round; they said they had my money, and so I let them in. I was getting their stuff for them, and one of them gets hold of my bag, waves it in my face and says "You're no getting it back, ya radge bitch."' She puts her hand to her mouth. 'Sorry, Doctor…'

Roxi curses freely in my presence. After a certain, arbitrary number of curses she does this thing, putting her fingers to her mouth, says 'Aw, sorry, Doc,' like I'm prone to offence, like I'm a vicar in a seventies sitcom.

But I'm getting the picture. Some men, associates of Jelly-Boy, have come to her house, where Roxi lives alone with no one but Coco, her Staffie, to give her some money in exchange for … goods?

'So one of them's got ma bag, and the other gets Coco by the collar, and he's twisting the collar, and wee Coco's making these … these *awful* honking noises…'

I nod. Quiet. I'm hooked by Roxi's story – I always am – and I need to know how it plays out. I'm also short of time, and Roxi's stories don't ever end. But I'm committed now. I nod. *And then?*

'It all started with a kiss…'

What?

'Well. Mebbe a wee nibble.'

I didn't used to like Roxi.

Not quite true. I *always* liked Roxi. It was more that I never felt quite *ready* for her. Certainly never had the time. Never quite *up for it*. She has chaos about her. She has something that is dangerous and uncontainable. I never know what she might say or do next. Her emotions are huge. I shy away from conflict while Roxi rises to it.

She thinks that I'm a dick – I think that's the word she used. Sometimes, unconsciously, when talking to me, I think she puts on *my* accent: soft, middle-class, educated east coast Scots. She does it uncomfortably well. This is what Roxi *really* thinks of me. True enough, she makes me sound like a dick.

At Christmas time she came in in tinsel and a battered little santa hat, stood at the reception desk and tried to lead a chorus of staff and patients in 'Shangalang': 'We sang Shangalang with the rest of the gang, singing shoobidoobidoobidooway…!' conducting with her finger tips and her flailing arms. 'Come on guys, sing-a-long, it's Christmas time!'

But there were people there with babies that weren't feeding and had temperatures, silent girls fading away because they wouldn't eat, old men with tumours in the throat that couldn't, a young man who lost his job because he turned up drunk one day, and another that didn't even know why he's there because he can't find the words to say. But people were coerced by Roxi's Potent Christmas Spirits, and a few even started to sing, mumbling along, ashamed of themselves for doing it, before I called her through early, to get her out of there, to put an end to the agony.

She is altogether *too much*. She calls me 'Darling!' She doesn't listen, and when I try to give her medical advice she just rolls her eyes and interrupts me with a story about her dog, or a man she once knew who was an Elvis impersonator that reminded her a little of me. 'Dr Dorward, do you ever sing in clubs? Because there's this man…' There are no gaps in her speech, no prosody at all, it's all content with Roxi, all fluctuating mood: sobs, tears, laughter.

Her face is cut and scarred from violent treatment at the hands of men. Her past is written on her face. Her face was stamped on when she was a young woman, and she has cooked her gums with the hot gases that she has been inhaling since childhood. Heroin and meth burn at a high temperature. If you inhale them, soon enough your teeth wobble, then fall out. Roxi has terrible teeth: those that she has remaining are crooked hooks and spikes for eating with, and biting. She has that closed mouth smile that people who have been stamped on use to hide the shameful fact of their damage. From time to time she asks me to refer her to a plastic surgeon to get her face sorted. Sometimes she asks me to refer her to a dentist. To my shame, until now I have just changed the subject, distracted her to something else, quite overwhelmed.

I have a *commitment* to liking her, which you might say isn't the same as saying I like her – but I think works well enough. It's the work we all have to do, to get along. It's like a lived vow, a faith, at times lived effortfully.

The truth – I'm ashamed to say – is that I'm also a little afraid of Roxi.

When I was a trainee, on my very last day of training in fact, I was attacked by a violent psychopath. I had seen this girl – a child, really, a waif – in the morning, and she had bothered me a lot. She was 17 or 18 and she was vomiting. Her new boyfriend had just got out of prison a month or so previously; he had been on remand for assault on a baby – someone else's baby – but had been found not guilty. The baby was in care now, somewhere, elsewhere, now safe. It was clear that his new girl was pregnant. With the boyfriend out of prison and her being sick a lot, it was an easy enough diagnosis, confirmed by two dots on the pee-strip. Even a year into this complex job, you can sometimes see what's coming from the moment the person walks in the door. Or at least you think you can.

She also had two bruises on her throat, one on each side of her trachea, unmistakably the size of two thumbs. Another easy diagnosis, but a great deal harder to deal with. Moving on from the news of the pregnancy (she was delighted, I wasn't), I tried to ask her about her bruises, but I was 20-something and had no skill, no experience of this kind of thing, and she was evasive anyway, didn't want to say anything, and so she left.

Later that afternoon, a man came to see me in his early thirties, Bic tattoos on his knuckles, with the same girl from earlier in tow, pale, thin-looking, bruises still livid on her pale throat. Her whip-strong, tobacco-breathed man, older than me, wanted something to control his mood swings. 'The last doctor gave me these,' he said, thrusting an empty strip of valium under my nose. I said maybe not, at which point the girl, the child, the waif, belligerent, came to his aid saying, 'So are you saying you won't help him then? Are you *refusing him the help he needs*?'

And I say, 'No, but…'

And she says, 'He's the same one I saw this morning…'

And he says, 'Ah telt ye, this is *such* a fucking waste of time.'

And I stand – to run? to reason? – and raise my voice a little, obviously getting angry, obviously frightened, but suppressing it. But he can smell it – he actually sniffed the air, like a hound, sniffed the fear. I saw him do it. I held up my hands, saying, 'Hang on a minute…'

And that was enough. The man had a chair in his hands, and he swung it. I hid under the desk. The girl ran away. I tried to find the emergency bell, couldn't, and then it didn't work. The chair broke on the desk. I shouted as loudly as I could. Someone else came into the room, saw what was happening, and ran away. Then the incident was over.

Not quite over.

Six months later I was working abroad. One of the perks of privilege is that you get to move on, you get to live as many lives as you please in the time you're given. I had pretty much forgotten the con with his prison tattoos and his child-like girl. I was working on a project to try to improve health facilities in communities of ex-combatants from Reagan's Nicaraguan war. Scotland seemed a long time ago. A gentle place; a soft, longed for place, far away. I had nipped out to buy a cold drink from the water seller in the street outside. I was spending the day in the office handwriting a fax, a project report, as I'd be returning to the field in a day or two. The secretary in the office I was borrowing held the phone up for me. This never happened. No one used to call me there.

'Es *la policia*! Escocesa!' She looked a little shocked.

It was a DCI Macmerry from Highland CID. He wanted to interview me over the phone, to get some details about an incident that had happened, shortly before I had left my last job. There had been a recent murder, and my story might be relevant collateral evidence. An infant, a baby girl, had been thrown against a brick wall in a flat in Inverness, and had died of head injuries. The child's mother, a teenager, was saying she didn't know what had happened, though the police knew she did. They suspected the father, who had previously been acquitted of something similar. It seemed that I had met him once.

I have no real call to be afraid of Roxi, none at all, but the child murderer from Inverness inoculated me with a prejudice. Whenever I met *his type* again I would re-experience that gooseflesh I had felt for a second or two as I hid under my desk. My heart would pound, my mouth would go dry, the skin on my hands too. I would sweat and my breath would come short and fast. I would find myself for a moment, back there, right back in that situation, afraid. Is that *really* a prejudice? Surely that's just good sense – just what anyone needs to survive in any world, even one as relatively benign as mine. But pretty soon my skin-crawling became overgeneralised. It wasn't just 30-something Scots men with knuckle tatts that got me like this, but pretty much anyone who carried with them a whiff of unpredictable rage and violence, the turbulent and the volatile, and that covers an awful lot of people. So whenever I met them – those crims and junkies, psychos, batterers, the violent, the bad – and those legions of their victims who were to me, it seemed, all just the same, my hypothalamus would go off like a fire bell, ringing fight or flight, and just as likely the former. I felt threatened, and just couldn't seem to hide it. If I were a soldier or an ambulance man or a policeman, I might think it was post-traumatic stress disorder, but it's not. In my case, it's just a prejudice.

As prejudices go, however, this one isn't disabling. Fearing, and then inevitably hating, this population is pretty socially acceptable. Normal, in fact. Encouraged, really, in some quarters at least. I think, or I would like to think, or my privilege allows me to think, that in my world to be overtly racist or sexist or hating of confessions distant from one's own, or to be hating of others whose sexualities one finds unappealing, would be hard. At the very least, it would become self-regulating. You would pretty soon learn to shut up about it, or you would earn a reputation for boorishness or ignorance. Not so a prejudice against violent, addicted crims. Generally speaking, that's fine. You would be mad not to fear *them*.

Once you know this in yourself, though, there are ways to manage. It's your fear that makes you vulnerable, and you can hide that behind a carapace of hard, binary rules. Try saying this, for example: *These are dishonest liars. Everything they say and do is part of a scheme. To get more drugs. A dishonest sick note. A moment alone in the office so that they can filch some blank prescriptions. Perpetrate some scam so unfathomable that it has no bottom. You just need to say no, pre-emptively and firmly.*

No. No!

You can say that *these people* are manipulative. They don't treat others – you, me – as people, but as objects, things in the world that they can manipulate for their benefit. You could argue that by seeking to use us, in a fundamental way they transgress a contract that exists between all of us – to treat one another as the same kind. They are *adults*, not children. They make their own decisions. By violating this basic contract, this fundamental rule of what it means to have a human relationship, they lose the right to be treated as a person. If they treat you as a thing, then you must treat them so. You might take this a little further. Emotional honesty is the material that imparts tensile strength to human relationships. Lose that honesty and relationships are just spun words and empty actions; they have no resilience. If you *pretend* respect, you trade in the same false currency of lies. This forms the beginnings of a rule. Something solid. Something reassuringly table-like, that you can hide under. No one will criticise you for applying hard binary rules. Consistency as an epistemological virtue straddles science *and* philosophy.

So, the people I am frightened of most, have a propensity to most violence. They are abusive. They shout and swear and kick off unpredictably and with a minimum of provocation. So we can all adopt a zero tolerance rule. You can even put a sign up in the waiting room and other public places in the surgery stating what kinds of behaviour will be tolerated. You can call the police when these rules are broken. You can apply hard, binary rules and can draw lines that mustn't be crossed. For example, these people are often late. They are disorganised and waste your time with irrelevancies. They often fail to turn up to appointments, wasting your time and everyone else's. So if they are late, you don't need to see them, and if they don't turn up at all, kick them off your list and make them find another doctor. And only ever deal with one problem at a time. If they have several, make them rebook. They rarely do.

These people know the law, or think that they do. They will often threaten to complain about you, loudly, publicly, seeking to intimidate you in order to get their way. If they have a complaint, you can insist on them writing it down. Most of them are illiterate, and so will be too ashamed to press it. In any case, they come and go, these folk. Most of the time their mobiles are either nicked or out of contract, so just try to contact them a few times. They won't answer, and if you can't contact them, then you can legitimately kick them off your surgery list.

With the application of hard rules, the problem pretty soon seems to go away. You end up seeing fewer hostile people. Life becomes a little easier. You can live in a world where these people don't impact. It seems to work pretty well in practice, at least from the doctor's point of view. If you give nothing away, then you won't be consumed.

I had a colleague once, years ago, called Margarita, who seemed quite unaffected by these problems. I could be critical at times of Margarita, and she of me, but I respected this: those

very people who most made me sweat, who most made me huff
and puff and strut like a hostile turkey, she seemed to have the
most cordial relationships with. Margarita, who was Greek,
came from an upper-class family of business people in Athens,
was educated at a private girls' school in England and *sang*
her vowels, never seemed to have trouble seeing the humanity in anyone, however unprepossessing. A lot of ordinary,
more highly functioning people found Margarita a little bit
aloof. Perhaps something about her cut-glass English grated
on a Scots ear. But not these special patients: her clientele of
broken people, the addicts, the scammers, the gaol birds, those
simmering with rage. She called them by their first names, and
they by hers.

'Hiya, Dr Margarita!'

'Roxanna, good morning. How is your dog?'

*'Muffy? He's deid. Had tae be pit doon. Ah've got a new one
though, he's called Coco.'*

*'Oh dear. I'm so sorry, Roxanna, but I'm sure Coco will be lovely.
Have you been shooting up heroin again?'*

'Me? Niver, just a wee ten pound burn bag, just tae keep me level.'

*'Oh dear … Oh well, never mind! Can we do a urine sample just
the same?'*

'Aye sure…'

I overheard a conversation once between Margarita and a man
called Tam. Tam was a rare thing. Tam was a heroin addict in
his mid-forties who still injected, and had done for more than
25 years, and yet was still alive. He was emaciated and broken,
yellow and tremulous with liver disease, dressed in rags, and
had no teeth. He smelled so bad that we sometimes had to see
him in a special room in the surgery.

'Hiya Margarita. Did ye have a nice holiday?'

'I did thank you, Tam.'

'*Were ye back in Greece, aye?*'

Tam had spent most of his adult life in prison. Mainly for shoplifting, but also a few years for GBH. Two drunk men squaring off to one another with blades ended badly, inevitably, and Tam got the blame.

'*Thank God you're back though, Dr Margarita. I had to see that Dr Dorward last month.*'

Tam was brought up in care. He looked very odd – runty and stunted, with sticky-out ears and a squint. He never really went to school. I think he's dead now.

'*He really looks down his nose at you … Looks at you as if you're pure shite…*'

I could be quite critical of Margarita, and she of me. But for some reason she had no need of my binary rules; no need for lines that couldn't be crossed.

———

The obligation to treat others always as an end, never as a means, seems rock solid when you apply it as a rule of thumb governing how you behave in the world, although it's hard at times to live up to. But it seems like a very high standard to apply to other people. The ability always to imagine others to be as real as oneself requires imaginative reach. It requires a high degree of social intelligence. It requires empathy. It requires you not only to understand about the reality of other people, it also requires you to *care*. That may not be too much to ask of you or me, but it is a lot to ask of everyone.

The principle of respect for autonomy is seen sometimes as the first among equals of ethical principles. Indeed it can be argued that those other principles with which it competes – an obligation to benefit people, an obligation to avoid harming them, a respect for justice – fold into respect for autonomy, and can be seen as subsidiary aspects to it. But autonomy, like all ethical principles, is social in nature. To be meaningful it has to contain within it the possibility of reciprocity. Does one have an obligation to respect the autonomy of a person who lacks the capacity to respect the autonomy of others? And if so, how far does this obligation extend?

Many of these people that trouble and frighten me have a degree of learning disability. Many have sustained brain injury through violence or chemicals or an accident of genes or birth. Almost all of them have extraordinarily poor emotional and social skills. The vast majority of the men have experienced violence as children at the hands of adults, and the vast majority of the women have experienced sexual abuse at the hands of men, and for those that haven't, that pattern of violence and sex is reversed. They have very little by way of social capital. In practice they are so rubbish at manipulation that their attempts to control, with words at least, can just seem laughable.

If you lack empathy, or social awareness, or deftness in language or manners, or if you are manipulative in your behaviour towards others, but bad at disguising it, you are about as socially impaired in our culture as it is possible to be. Those people who resort to violence to get what they want are, I think, on the extreme end of this spectrum of deficit. If access to medical care is, or, rather, should be, determined by need, then I have few patients as deserving of care as Tam.

———

You can always make funny stories from these situations, at least afterwards. The most painful ones are the best. I made a funny story out of Tam and Margarita and the overheard conversation, at least after a little time had passed. I shared it widely to colleagues, friends, students. There is inherent story material in the overheard conversation, in which the listener hears some unwelcome truth about himself, has his massive ego punctured by someone more humble than he is, then has to go home and think again.

There is nothing funny about Snakey McShane.

He is thin and lizard-like, with jet black hair combed back in a quiff. He wears fake reptile-skin boots and skinny jeans, denim shirt and sports a Texan hat that he lays upon the desk when he takes his ease in the chair opposite mine. There is nothing *ha ha ha* about Snakey. The air crackles around him. The temperature drops when he enters the room. His name is fake. Obviously. He leans back in the chair, and folds his arms upon his chest, waiting, bored. He has a tattoo, perhaps some glyph carved between his eyebrows a long time ago, which might just be a gravel rash from an accident he had as a young man, or just a deep wrinkle or indentation between his eyes. Or perhaps it's a cross, a swastika even. You don't ever want to look too close. You don't want to look too deeply into Snakey's black eyes. You look at him, then you look away, and he counts it as a tiny victory. You look too long into his little eyes and something snaps tight shut behind you.

'So, Mr McShane, how can I help?'

I sit up and a little forward. My arms are open and my body posture is relaxed. Posture is important in establishing rapport. I note my intense emotional reaction to this man – a little fear, irritation at his arrogance, his languorous and serpentine pose – and understand, as I have learned to understand, that my reaction to him is a *symptom*. That is to say, if this man makes me feel this way, this is probably how he makes everyone feel. So, Snake is surrounded by people in life who are frightened of him and a little irritated. This tells me something important about this man, his nature, his problem, his way of being – something that will emerge during the course of the conversation that we are about to have.

Stung by what I had overheard between Tam and Margarita, I went on a course – sent myself on it, before someone else felt they had to suggest it. A series of workshops looking at practical compassion. The course was brilliant. It was led by a charismatic, gentle, retired GP, who had clearly seen and experienced every-thing, and who suggested the idea (new to me) that the exercise of compassion was a practical skill – an example of wisdom in practice, a fundamental behaviour that could be learned and promoted. There was a little theory, a little talk of Aristotle and human flourishing, the virtues, and the nature of practical wisdom, but mainly it was about doing. How to sit, how to talk, how to ask questions, in such a way as to create a space between you and your patient, where kindness might flourish.

'I need something to help me to sleep.'

'Right.'

We have no records for Snakey. He registered the previous week, had seen the practice nurse for a checkup but refused to answer any of her questions, choosing instead to be glib: 'I prefer to be addressed as Reverend.' We know nothing about him, other than that he has changed his name, lives in a homeless hostel around the corner and smells strongly of rolling tobacco. The practice nurse was sufficiently concerned to warn me: 'There's something not right about him.'

Too right. But I suppress the shudder and the desire to just give him what he wants and get him out. If I behave in a certain way, model a certain way of being, it creates the environment where some kind of mutual respect can, in time, occur. Get away from the application of hard rules. Acknowledge your fear, irritation, prejudice towards this man, then put it to one side. Find the humanity.

'Why can't you sleep?'

He pauses for a moment or two. His arms are folded in front of him. He has a little smile playing on his lips. He looks at me through narrowed, flickering black eyes. I look away, again. There should be something funny about this whole cowboy shtick. There just isn't.

'Because whenever I shut my eyes I see in my head the face of a wee princess.'

Eh?

'And the face of the man that killed her. So I cannae sleep.' He waits for my response. He has all day. I don't. I sense very strongly that he knows this. The disparity between my time and his is leverage.

It feels like a physical effort to ask him: 'Whose face is it that you see?'

'My granddaughter.'

According to his date of birth, he is in his late fifties. Most men get fat as they age, but he hasn't. He has a lean, hard, lined look to him. He has clearly told this story many, many times before. It is as if he can barely raise the emotional capital to be bothered to tell it all again. That is to say, he seems *bored*.

'So your wee girl, your granddaughter, was killed and now you can't sleep?'

'Aye. Oh, and …' And as if an afterthought, '… I need a sick note too.'

'What's on the sick note?'

'Depression. And insomnia.'

Later, I do a thing I almost never do. I check out his story. There was an old news article on Google, and there was a picture of Snakey, the tell-tale smudge between his eyebrows identifying him as no other, even though his name was changed, performing (but why *performing*?) the role of the bereaved grandfather. The girl, a 14 year old, was sleeping in alleys. She had an eating disorder, and was an alcoholic. Her boyfriend, who was much, much older, a man in his thirties, also an alcoholic, had given her some spirits and some pills, 'to help her to sleep' he had said in his defence, but, rendered unconscious, she had vomited, and he had found her frozen, dead on a bench the next morning. The man, also pictured, who squinted into the camera lens, glassy eyed, haggard, sad and broken, said that he had loved her, said that he had tried CPR but didn't know how to do it, went down for manslaughter. The younger Mr McShane, according to the article, was going to sue social services for neglecting his wee princess. I don't know whether he did. I don't know whether he won.

My hand was shaking a little as I signed a prescription for valium, 30 milligrams a day, enough to stun an ox.

But later I thought *Where were* you *when the child was drinking herself to sleep?*

Under the pressure of the moment, I wrote him a sick note, wrote 'depression and insomnia', feeling as I did that I was perpetrating a fraud.

But later I thought *Where were you when she was taken into care? What help did* you *offer when she sought solace in the company of this man who poisoned her?*

Whenever I sign these documents it is as if a little more is chipped away from my integrity. It is as if a tiny little bit of what is good and honest in the world is diminished. Snakey placed the documents in the pocket of his skinny jeans.

But later I thought *At least the man who killed her* tried *to love her.*

He gets up to leave. I can't just leave it at that though. I can't bring myself to practise medicine at this terrible level of crapiness. I can't be that doctor – although in this man's case there must be a whole long line of us – who just signs the prescription and sick note and sighs a sigh of relief to see the back of him.

I say, 'Make an appointment as you go. I'll see you in a month.'

He raises an eyebrow. *Why?*

'Let's see if we can do anything more to help with your insomnia. And your … depression.'

He shrugs his shoulders, smirks, doesn't even bother to respond. Leaves.

I rant to my friend.

I rant a lot to my friend, who is generous with his time, and not easily bored. We go on long runs together on the hill just behind where we live. Hard exercise is cleansing of all the crap one can accumulate during the practice of medicine.

I say, 'It's not so much that he's bad. I see a lot of bad people. I know a thing or two about bad people…'

Thomas grunts. It's still dark and raining lightly. Thomas is younger and much fitter than I am. He is opening some distance between us on the slippery steps. Eight switch backs on the steep bit, then the path levels out onto a plateau. I struggle to catch up.

'… and I'm sure that his mum and dad were horrible to him. I'm sure that he was battered from here to breakfast time, but I just cannot make myself pretend to like this man.'

There are 10 yards between us now. I'm slipping and staggering, yelling and ranting, all at once.

'He *uses* his dead granddaughter … he uses her as leverage … it's like it's his income…'

Thomas waits for me on the level. We round the corner of the first summit, find ourselves in the shadow of the wind, and we can see the first light of sunrise in the east by Berwick Law.

'… But the thing that I *really* hate…'

Thomas grunts and picks up speed again, but I catch him easily. I'm warmed up now, really in my stride.

'… The thing that I really hate is that being *nice* to him just seems to add fuel to his malevolence. My attempt at kindness is just *currency* for him.' I pause, out of breath. 'Fuck compassion,' I say, bitterly.

For a magical moment, as we stand there, sweating and out of breath, we are both illuminated by a pink glow. There is a dark lid of thick cloud, low over the sky, but it is clear in the east, and the first sun shines under the cloud. Blue sky in the east, rosy sunlight, dark bruised clouds overhead.

Thomas says, or at least I think he says because there's a light breeze blowing away his words and he mumbles, 'We're all God's children,' and takes off again like a hare, scurrying up the narrow path to the summit, damp rock now glistening in early sunlight.

That is not, at all, the kind of thing that Thomas would say, unless he was taking the piss, which is totally possible. Thomas has first-class degrees in just about everything, as well as medicine. 'We're all God's children' isn't at all the kind of facile comment he would make, unless he was really desperate to end the conversation. I don't even know if Thomas believes in God at all, although I suspect he doesn't.

I've never found appeals to God helpful in settling questions of should or shouldn't. Either God tells us that things are good because they are independently good, in which case he is in the same game as we are of interpretation of what is good and what isn't, only his argument is less clearly and succinctly expressed, or he is asserting that a thing is good because he says it is, in which case his assertion is arbitrary and the argument empty.

On the other hand, the phrase does have some rhetorical force. I repeat it to myself as I slow to a very slow pace on the steep, last section. I take the direct route, hands and feet in play as I scramble up damp crags. On the face of it, this is the bolder route to the top, but since the birth of his children, Thomas won't take it, fearing a fall. I berate him for his cowardice. In any case, I think he's wrong. It's the slippery steps that are lethal. Hands and feet carefully placed on the rock, attention absolutely focused, nothing much is going to go wrong.

'We are all God's children.' I like the solidarity expressed in that. I like the grandeur and the simplicity. I could imagine myself using that phrase for real.

Thomas at the top is scarcely out of breath. We share a smile. It is proper daylight now.

'Did you say what I thought you said, down there?'

'What?'

'Did you say, "We are all God's children"?'

Thomas looks at me with the same skeptical *are you stupid?* look that he has directed at me since he was about 10, and that his four-year-old has already started to adopt.

'No, course not,' and starts off running again, heading back down for breakfast.

We are all God's children.

Roxi said: *It started with a kiss.*

'I was only joking around, at least at first. But he's got my bag and he's waving it around saying "Is that where yi've got Jelly-Boy's money!" But there was no money in that bag. There was never any money in that bag, but Coco … Coco's always looked after me. Coco bites him, just a wee nip, just a nibble really, so his pal, he gets Coco's collar and pulls, and Coco's making this terrible honking noise, so he throws the bag back down and shouts "Christ, ye can have yer bag back, ye auld boiler." And ah ken that if Jelly-Boy wisnae in the gaol he wid never, *niver* have said that, he'd be too feart, and so I say, "I'll fucking boil *ye!*" And I grab him, and suddenly it's like I'm going to kiss him, although I widnae kiss him really because of Jelly-Boy, I wid niver do that. Although he's my ex, I'll always be faithful. It would kill him. But I still grab him, more like a hug, and he tries to kiss *me*, but my tooth catches him on the nose, like. See this tooth? It caught him on the nose, and he tries to pull away and it's like Ah've torn it off…'

She points to the remains of a tooth.

'Ah can still feel his skin where it snagged, it's disgusting…'
Right.

'And you know the funny thing, Doctor? When the police get there, they look in my bag, and do you know what they find?'
No.

'They find £115! God knows where it came from. I think they gave me my money after all! From Jelly-Boy.'

'What happened to the man you … kissed?'

'He'll be okay. They sewed it back on. He's in the hospital. Says he doesn't want to press charges, but the police say they've got to.'

'Have you been to prison before?'

'Aye. It's not prison that's bothering me. It's wee Coco. That dog's been everything to me. It's not *his* fault. He's been like a *husband* to me. Not like *that*, obviously, but … gentle.

Soft as a feather, sweet as a flower. Just like a husband ought to be.'

She looked at the floor, eyes filling again with tears.

———

So, to conclude, some rules of thumb for dealing with people you fear:

+ Nurse your compassion – it's finite. Be flexible in its application.
+ Make up soft, pragmatic rules, but don't be too afraid to break them.
+ Find the humanity – we're all God's children, after all.
+ Let the conversation take you where it will, but keep close to the door.
+ Be honest. Never, ever lie.

———

'So what happened to Coco?'

'They put him in a kind of cage. It was like the man from the animal welfare was frightened of him. It was like he was frightened of *me*. He's saying all this shit, that they'd look after him and stuff, but then they put him in a cage and, even though they've sedated him, Coco's going mental! It was like they were frightened of him. It was like they were frightened of *me*. It was like they couldn't get out of there fast enough. Why were they frightened of *me*? What'll they do with Coco, Doctor, if I go to prison?'

I shake my head, and lie. 'I don't know.'

'He's such a good dog…' She's getting up to leave, at last.

And this is the point at which, feeling *terribly sorry* for Roxi, and for Coco, and for all the sadness that there is in the world, I say, 'You'll be okay...' and put my hand on her elbow, and she says 'Aye, right,' and shakes my hand off.

So we stand there for a moment or two, she leaving, my waiting for her to go. Then she says, 'Can you do me a letter, d'ye think, Doctor? For Coco, not for me, for the animal welfare. Can *you* tell them that he's a good dog? Can you write it so that they don't put him down?'

And I, running half an hour late, desperate to finish, say, 'Yes. I will. Of course I will,' lying, again.

And then Roxi leaves, for prison, I'm sure.

Three Views of a Mountain

Years pass, and now I can scarcely believe some of the things I did, the ways in which I thought, the risks that I took, the things that I believed to be true. I can't quite credit how much things change. Almost everything that I see in my clinic now is a variation on a pattern, a new reading of something that I have seen before. Days go by and nothing is entirely new. Different circumstances, different outcomes, but the same key plots: same drives, same jeopardies.

When I was starting out, each problem I saw seemed new, each tiny thread of its complex weave to be run to its source. It took forever. It killed me. I could never see the overall shape of things. I was like a child learning to read, spelling out the names of things from their individual letters, stumbling endlessly over individual words whilst the text flowed beyond me. Now I read whole sentences at a glance.

When a person consults with me now, I can sometimes see the outcome after only a few words. Sometimes I can read a person's story in the movement of their body as I greet them: they stand, and I think *I know this one! I know how this story goes*. That doesn't make things dull. My days are never dull. In fact, it adds fascination. I see things in a finer grain. It gives texture and detail. It brings with it this new delight: of finding oneself to be *experienced* and, during one's better days, an *expert*, even.

Before, confronted with a difficult new patient, I sometimes felt like a stone falling down a well. The uncertainty felt sudden, total and overwhelming; it drowned me. The isolation felt like darkness closing. Sometimes I feel that now, but it's rarer. Back then, a young woman, for example, might open her mouth and tell me that she was cutting herself, her wrists and her thighs, with a pencil sharpener, every night, and she would raise her sleeves and show me these thin, pink parallel stripes, and there I would be, falling down a deep well, thinking *What can I possibly say to her that will help? What can I possibly do?* I feared that I would have nothing to offer, nothing at all, and that always seemed so terrible.

This morning Jodie, a patient, comes to see me again, angry as hell – always angry – saying that, because I tried to reduce the dose of her Valium, she had done *this*. And she yanks up her sleeve and thrusts her sliced forearms into my face, and asks what was I going to do? Jodie's great-uncle is also her father. She has the ghost of a memory from her childhood that he might have been more than that, too. But her mother, who is dead now, would never talk about it (who would?) and she's not speaking to her aunties or her sisters, so that leaves Jodie thrusting her wounds into her doctors' faces, her own face twisted into a *fuck you* shriek. And I say to Jodie that there is nothing that I *can* do, because there isn't, and that seems less terrible to me now, than it did, before. Because I have seen hundreds of people who cut.

Because I have seen so many cases, I have a mantra for people who cut. The same mantra I use for all my patients whose faces carry that look, the patients who invoke from my depths the ghost of that same shriek.

Jodie looks at me through narrowed, angry eyes.

Slowly, I breathe in my mantra; slowly I breathe it out:

+ *De-escalate.* Reduce the emotional charge – mine and theirs. Be calm.
  Pause, breathe deeply. I don't show desperation or impatience; I don't show anger, with the world, or its victims. Suppress it all. I don't glance at my watch. I don't prescribe impulsively, I don't refer impulsively, I don't do anything that raises the emotional temperature. I'm calm. I'm present. I reassure.

+ *Be honest.* Say it as it is: cutting is common. With calm and reassurance, with time, it usually passes. Your personality is as it is, and I can't fix that, because it is you. This cutting is your thing, not mine, but I will try to help you to find a better way through. There isn't a drug or a therapy or a person that will *make* you stop. Any cheap solution is a lie, and I won't offer it. But I will try to help.

+ *Be there.* I will be here for a long time. For as long as I am here, I will be happy to see you. I will try to be available, I will remember who you are, and I will still try hard to care. I will try to build a relationship with you even when no one else will. I hope to be the last person standing when everyone else is gone.

Now that I have seen how common it is, it doesn't panic me so, when I discover that people cut themselves to deal with pain. Silent, I breathe in the mantra, breathe it out.

'Why did you cut yourself *today*, Jodie?'

———

And then it is Thursday afternoon, my favourite time of the week – the springtime of the week, when the sun comes out at last and the flowers bud. I get to teach the FY2s. An FY2 is a new doctor, qualified for just one year. There are six of them in my group, all young women in their mid to late twenties, well educated, fiercely motivated, from all over, but a narrow demographic nonetheless. They file in, chatting, and sit around my room in a clutter of shoulder bags. Confident women. I delegate the one I know best to make the tea; one opens a plastic box of homemade biscuits. One of the countless benefits of the feminisation of medicine that has taken place over the last 25 years or so is that doctors are better, in almost all respects, than they used to be. Another is the vast improvement in the quality of the baking.

'What's that?' asks one, gesturing to a picture on my wall.

Three Views of a Mountain.

Three representations, arranged vertically. A conical shape, possibly Mount Fuji. The first representation, the topmost, is applied in thick oils, all reds, blacks, oranges, and is the fiery representation. The second, the middle of the two, is a watercolour. A sense of spring time, imparted by green on the lower slopes, a patch of pale blue for water at the foot of the mountain, sail boats blown like petals across the shoreline, a clear sky, few clouds. The third, at the bottom, is a single calligraphic brush stroke in black, representing the form of the volcano, its cupped summit, and beside it, in red ink, a Japanese symbol, for 'peace', or 'understanding', or 'sympathy'.

'It's...' *one of my most precious possessions,* I realise, in the moment of opening my mouth, ignorant until that instant of how much that picture means to me. 'It's a present. It was a present from a patient. A long time ago.'

She would be a qualified doctor now. She would be a consultant psychiatrist, or maybe a GP. Perhaps she has kids. It was such a long time ago. Name signed in pencil at the bottom. Jemma. Jemma Borderas.

My students pause, looking at it, considering the simplicity of its form, the contrasts, the worlds contained within it, the simple flourish of talent that made it.

———

I first met Jemma Borderas when she was a junior medical student. She was one of a group of three. We piled into my car and drove around the corner to the house of an old woman, a decaying, smart, rich, arty lady, who lived in antique splendour in a mews flat in Pimlico and was dying of heart failure. We stood, the four of us, in the shadows cast around her tiny truckle bed edged into tight spaces by monumental acts of furniture and the housekeeper brought us tea.

I ask the first, a boy of twenty-something, to feel her pulse and ask him what he might find in the pulse in such a case, thinking as I do how much I correspond to my own image of Victorian doctor-teacher. I catch a glimpse of myself in a wardrobe mirror in my dark suit, leaning attentively over the dying woman's bed, the heavy quilted blankets, the sick-bed smell of sweat and urine. I look like my grandfather.

The boy looks blank, as the boys did then, and have done always.

'Rate?' I suggest.

'Fast, irregular…' he says, flustered.

'Good.'

I ask the next to look at the old woman's neck, to check the venous pulse, elevated in heart failure, hard to see in the shadows. He lifts the old woman's chin without first asking her, and I gently chastise him, 'Always ask before touching,' and think *that's a good lesson to learn.*

'Jemma?' I look up, looking for the girl, but she isn't there. 'Jemma?'

Jemma's drifted off. Like a child, Jemma's lost interest and has drifted to the opposite side of the room, where she is inspecting a wall, covered side to side and top to bottom in Japanese-style prints. Jemma has long black hair, streaked with henna. She wafts tobacco, sweat and patchouli. She has lines of studs in her left ear, and when she talks there is the flash of a tongue piercing. Tiny mouse-like Jemma wears a long pencil skirt and tight black t-shirt, vest style, cut low, which shows a little rosebud tatt above her right breast. The chaps wear shirts and ties. In the world of medicine, Jemma's style is *completely* inappropriate.

'Jemma?'

Not Japanese *style* prints, *real* prints. Real. Yellowed paper. The smell of age. Colours vigorous still, all in ink. Tigers. Dragons. Bridges with figures, men and women carrying kindling over tottering twig-like structures, waves and sunsets, boats with sails, a flash of red calligraphy, a view over water to a volcano.

'*Jemma!*'

This is funny, but embarrassing too. Although Mrs Bostyon is as old as time and wheezing out her last breaths, and although she is demented and in the care of her dodgy housekeeper, we are, nonetheless, her guests. This is *her* bedroom.

'Jemma, could you please listen to Mrs Bostyon's chest, and tell me what you think you can hear?'

She pulls herself away from the enchanted wall, back into this gloomy place and the gloomy present day, and says, 'I haven't got my stethoscope.' Jemma has a bit of an accent: South-East London, second-generation immigrant. The two boys with their shirts and ties and black cardiology stethoscopes hanging from their necks roll their eyes.

'Borrow mine!' I say.

Twenty years later and six female doctors sit around a table, none wearing inappropriate dress, none with visible tatts, none with implausibly coloured hair, no piercings other than a single pearl sitting in the earlobe, none with anything but the politest voice in the class. The demographic of doctors has narrowed. Each has her stethoscope in her shoulder bag. All are prepared.

Epidemics of Social and Culture-Bound Illness … is today's topic.

'Anyone do the reading?'

I set my bar of expectation low, but needn't. Nowadays, *everyone* has *always* done the reading. Doctors and medical students are selected to be the sorts of people who have always done the reading. No more *Jemmas* these days. Not a chance. No more callow young men with spots and bad attitudes either, who *just scrape through* and would never, ever, do the reading. No me, in other words.

There is a ducking of heads and a murmur of assent. They have all done the reading.

'Thoughts?'

There is a moment or two of silence (there always is) before someone talks. The trick is for me not to break that silence myself. If I break that silence, I will talk for two hours. My voice will drone: it will be like the despairing deep buzz of a huge mansplaining fly butting its head against the window glass as it tries to escape into the cold, free air outside. Mobile devices will be unsheathed, half concealed below the table lip, but I will still know that they are there.

I raise my eyebrows; I keep my silence.

The reading is an article from *The New Yorker* magazine, by a journalist called Rachel Aviv that I'd emailed around a few days earlier, given to me by my Scandi sister-in-law: 'Uppgivenhetssyndrom. Resignation Syndrome'. It is about an epidemic confined entirely to refugee children in Sweden, who have been denied leave to remain in the country. It occurs mainly amongst bilingual children who have entirely identified with their host culture, but who face deportation with their families because their parents fail to pass increasingly strict rules governing who in Sweden now qualifies for refugee status. Affected children become indolent; they stop talking, take to their beds, and stop eating or drinking. They are fed through tubes: an advocate for the children says get them tubed early because that way they will lose less muscle bulk and get less ill. The feeding tube will confirm their diagnosis and enable the care and benefits that they need to survive *and*, what's more, enable the possibility of recovery. Recovery results, in all cases, when the threat of deportation is lifted. It is evidently inhuman to deport a child dependent on a feeding tube. The article is headed by a picture of two adolescent Kurdish sisters, side by side in bed, their hair spread across their pillows, with the article referring to them in a slightly off-key way as 'angelic'. The doctor/advocate, Dr Hultcrantz, drives from end to end to the remotest parts of her long country because, in Sweden, refugees are resettled in small communities to try to prevent the creation of ghettos, and to promote integration. She works in her own time, unpaid, fighting for health provision, benefits, legal appeals, for her affected children. I have the clearest image of her in my mind, although there is no photo: tired, humble, committed, striking, battle fatigued, *shaming*.

'Your thoughts on Uppgivenhetssyndrom?'

'The *Daily Mail* would love this. I can just see the headline…'

'Are these children *faking* it?'

'Could they be? Could *you*? Fake starving yourself half to death? Fake dehydration? Renal failure? Muscle wasting? Pressure sores? That's more than *faking it*.'

In my whole medical life, I think I have scarcely seen one person whom I thought, in the end, was truly, deliberately, faking it.

I say: 'Every illness has a cause, and epidemics have many causes. What are the *vectors* for malaria?'

'Poverty.'

'Standing water.'

'Mosquitos.'

'What are the vectors for "resignation syndrome"?'

'It's not the same thing. It's a behaviour, not an illness…'

'Imagine if a behaviour *could* be an illness. What then would be the vectors for this one?'

Silence.

'Come on!'

Despite my springtime Thursday optimism, I am a little tetchy today. I don't usually say 'come on!' with that edge in my voice to these formidably clever, organised women, but something has unsettled me. Just before my tutorial was due to start, the Jodie thing blew up. Jodie, sexually abused by the men in her family since early childhood, and a punch bag for their friends since maturity, is on a prescription of Valium, opiates, sedative anticonvulsants, antidepressants and methadone. Her drugs regimen is hateful, toxic and somehow inevitable. It has been my quixotic mission to rationalise it: to save Jodie at least from the *medical* abuse that scars her. She keeps herself on a level by smoking cannabis: she reeks of weed, she stinks out my surgery room. No single doctor has determined that she be on this cock-tail – enough to sedate a rugby team – but when any single doctor tries to reduce, or rationalise, or straighten it out, she responds with self-aggression. She cuts. She strings herself up and is cut down. She drinks poison. She ends up in emergency rooms, where she is given more, different sedatives. The thing is, though, I have found out that she isn't *actually* taking these tablets. On a pretext, I checked her spit for toxicology the last time I saw her. She *is* taking street heroin, but the Valium, and the opiates we prescribe, no. The sedative anticonvulsants that go for a fiver a strip in the dens around my work? No. And that suggests she's selling what I prescribe in order to buy heroin. Or food. Or stuff for her kids. Where I work, this is a common economic model.

I phoned the chemist, who knows me by my voice, and stopped her prescription. *How could I not?* So Jodie pitched up in my emergency slot, packing her new boyfriend and a lifetime of rage, ready for an argument, which I wasn't having.

'Go away,' I said, when she started shouting. All my stupid complacency, all my thoughts of that *stupid* mantra, out the window now. 'I won't be shouted at...'

'But what about her pain?' asked the boyfriend, yellow skinned, a broken reed with a mouth like a graveyard and a kind of orange- and maroon-coloured plastic shell suit that I haven't seen worn for years.

'Yeah! What about my *pain*? My fucking *depression*?' said Jodie, standing now, waving her arms around, making for the door, painlessly, and I say, losing it, '*Pain* is not your problem!' and Jodie says, 'What do *you* know about my *pain!*' and stomps out.

The vectors determining Jodie's *behaviour* might include the following:

+ Poverty;
+ Incest;
+ Violence;
+ Lack of education and no social provision for those with poor educational prospects;
+ Available repertoire of *self-harming* behaviours;
+ No simple-to-access easy-to-do work;
+ A culture of casual opiate, benzodiazepine and cannabis consumption prevalent in her demographic;
+ Me. Doctors who prescribe for her. Doctors like me.

And this last makes me feel wretched.

'Come on! What are the vectors for Resignation Syndrome?' I ask my students, suppressing an odd cocktail of hateful and irrelevant thoughts like:

I can't stand people like Jodie.
Somehow I have let Jodie down. I have betrayed her.
I hate conflict.
All the time and care spent on people like Jodie is time wasted. I'd be better off doing something else. I've always thought that I'd make a good violinist. Or a florist, perhaps.

A slight pause, and then the boldest says, 'Kindness. It's like *kindness* is the cause. The Swedish state prides itself on its compassion, and its openness to outsiders and refugees. This behaviour couldn't flourish anywhere else. No one would even notice.'

Jemma the medical student came to see me, in my role this time as doctor, not teacher. It was a long time ago since I'd last seen her, but I remembered her. I was surprised and pleased to see her. Jemma was a terrible student. Her head was always somewhere else. She didn't seem to know a thing about medicine. She was aloof. She had a slight arrogance towards her fellow students, affecting disdain for their narrowness, gender and privilege, in a flagrantly compensatory attempt to disguise the fact that she was struggling herself and didn't know who or what she was, or why she was there. She was quite unable to express these thoughts. She was too child-like still to cut it in an adult world. The other students just ignored her.

I remembered Jemma, because when *I* was a student I fancied myself a bit of a poet. Bit aloof. Bit unpopular. Bit of a creative artist. Was always doing shows: playing *Puck!* In the *nude!* I was always failing exams, always scraping through. It wasn't until I was about 23 that I could reliably have a clean shirt ready for the morning, but ironing was still years off. I remember with fondness those kind adults who saw through me, and still cared. Something about Jemma's low-level squalor rang a bell.

She looks tired, hungover, washed out, pale, wan, tiny, thin, still in her black t-shirt with long sleeves and leggings, her clothes not altogether fresh.

'My tutor thinks I must have ME or depression or something.'

I don't say anything.

'She asked me to come. *She* thinks that's what it is…'

I sigh.

'Do you think you've got it?'

'I don't know. What *is* ME?'

For Jemma, it started with glandular fever, a month or two prior. She hadn't really properly recovered. She felt washed out. She was tired all the time. Couldn't be bothered to get up. Couldn't be bothered with her friends or flatmates. Didn't really know if she wanted to do medicine any more. She was assailed by headaches and body aches and a desire that would seize her at any time of day or night to sleep, for hours. She had tried going home for a few days, but her parents, who wanted her to work in their cafe, and couldn't bear her nocturnal habits, had eventually kicked her out. Her mood, she said, was fine.

Working in a university town, I saw a lot of students like that: people whose lives were overgrown with indolence. Knotweed. Clever, talented people, people who had worked hard, or whose parents had worked hard for them, who would attend some kind of elite institution of science, or medicine, art, or music, and would do okay for a bit, but who would slow down, engines clogged and sputtering. They would stop attending, stop working, fail exams, take to their beds, become powerless to rescue themselves. They would attract diagnoses, if they ever came to anyone's attention: they were told they were depressed, or drinking too much, taking too many drugs. They might latch on to an illness for a while, or get a label, like anxiety or post-viral fatigue. Sometimes, mostly, they would disappear, because the institution that first noticed that they were failing would lose patience with them, and then they would be gone. I used to see it all the time, this symptom pool … whatever it was. For a long time, it never really had a name. Then it did.

'It *feels* like I just can't be arsed anymore.'

Can't be arsed. Definitely not a legitimate diagnosis. I feel myself falling into a well, clawing for purchase on its slippery sides.

Why not ME? It was the nineties after all. The diagnosis was everywhere. Pervasive tiredness, unrefreshing sleep, low exercise tolerance, muscle pain, no primary mood disorder, a world of theories about the cause, with nothing proven. I can't remember what the diagnostic criteria for ME were then – they've changed – but she definitely met them, and even if she didn't quite, she might have had its *forme fruste*, its incomplete form, a borderline case? The distinction is arbitrary: the diagnosis is by assertion, either by the patient, or by the patient conforming to some diagnostic criteria, which themselves are rhetorical. It's not something in nature that you either *have*, or *don't*.

Her bloods, checked a week or two earlier by a colleague, were all fine, and that's always the case with ME. If a test is positive, the ailment stops being ME and becomes whatever the test says it is: a thyroid imbalance, or leukaemia, or diabetes, or glandular fever, or any of the infinite range of illnesses that might present in their first stage as unfathomable tiredness. Tiredness being a symptom, not a disease.

'Are you managing to do anything that you enjoy?'

'Meh…,' she says, evasive and irritating. But she has charcoal on her fingertips that I notice for the first time, and that gives me an obscure kind of hope. *Why are her fingers black?*

'We have to call it something. *Can't be arsed* absolutely doesn't count. If we don't have an explanation, the medical school will kick you out.'

Jemma shrugs her shoulders.

'Maybe you *are* depressed, and just don't know it?'

And maybe I wasn't quite *that* clumsy. Maybe I tested the water, waited a bit, before grabbing for that one. Maybe I raised one eyebrow in the quizzical doctor manner, echoed *can't be arsed eh?* and waited for the silence to be filled, for my patient to take me to the money...

Maybe I *was* more skilled then, than I remember, because I must have been, because Jemma came back to see me quite a few times, over the years. I must have said *something* helpful on that first day? Or maybe not. Maybe, glancing at my watch, getting annoyed with Jemma's hostile indifference, my need for a diagnosis and her inability to present with something *legitimate*, maybe I *was* that clumsy.

'*Maybe...*' said Jemma, unhelpfully.

Things I came to know about Jemma: she was the daughter of migrants. Her father owned a Catalan restaurant in Ilford and her mother was a doctor's receptionist. She had gone to a local comprehensive school, where her grades hadn't quite been good enough for medicine. She'd got in on her art portfolio. She'd won a national award for her A-level art, and that made her special enough to get in. That had swung it for Jemma. She had done well enough to get through her first couple of years at medical school in the lower middle of her class, but the trajectory of her grades was always earthward.

I asked her questions, she said 'Meh'. I crammed her symptoms into a box labelled 'depression'. A big, capacious box, right enough, but she still didn't altogether fit – bits kept popping out, limbs here and there, like stuffing a corpse into a suitcase – but eventually she all fitted in and I prescribed for her. Fluoxetine (Prozac), 20mg daily. A few words (too few) about side effects, delay in onset of action, duration of prescribing, arrangements made for review, all done in about 20 minutes.

'We don't see Resignation Syndrome in this country, although we will if the conditions are ever right for it to flourish. But we *do* see a lot of behaviours that we describe as illness. Behaviours evolve and, like everything that evolves, they exist in a niche. The niche for Resignation Syndrome is created by a refugee crisis, a country with a strong ethos of compassion and belonging, and, I think, a reaction to that: a country that is also riven with a new xenophobia and fear of outsiders. It's an illness of poor people in a wealthy country. It's a political illness. These are some of the factors that make Resignation Syndrome possible now in Sweden. Do we have any similar behaviours that are described as illness in this country?'

They look at one another, they look at me, they say nothing.

Sometimes it's important to be able to let the silence just sit. It's the discomfort of that silence that prompts words.

I let my eyes rest on the wall, at my *Three Views of a Mountain*. The angry view. The peaceful view, with its scattered boats and springtime watercolours. The brush stroke glyph at the bottom, and whatever its symbol means. Peace. Wisdom. Compassion. The passing of time.

I break the silence.

'ME? Chronic fatigue syndrome?'

There is little recognition. That slightly guilty look that doctors wear when they feel they *should* know about something.

'Does anyone know anything about that? Anyone? Chronic fatigue syndrome? ME?'

'Is that that post-viral thing?'

'My aunt had it! She was in a wheelchair for a few years. She's got dementia now.'

'But it's psychological, isn't it?'

'I don't know … is it even *real*?'

'Real? A real … *what*?'

I ask them, 'Would you ever diagnose it?' and they look at me as if I have asked whether they would ever make a diagnosis of the evil eye. Then the oldest one, the one that did an arts degree before going into medicine, the one whom I increasingly rely on to get things going, Klara, says, 'It's just a label – but with a lousy prognosis and no treatment. The only thing that you can offer for it is CBT, and that only works on the subgroup of patients who were going to get better anyway. The factor that most determines a negative outcome in ME is the degree of commitment to the diagnosis. It's like the name itself carried the plague. Why would I make *that* diagnosis? No one wants it any more. It's a life sentence.'

But now the epidemic is disappearing. For 20 years it was a staple of talk shows and newspaper articles. It was a topic of conversation and everyone who was involved was angry about it. Now, in my experience, people just don't present with it, and for people who are tired all the time – and there are just as many of these as ever – we don't offer it as an explanation. As Klara says, it's like the label itself carried the plague.

Klara, again: 'It was like a *social metaphor*. I think it was a metaphor for AIDS. It started at about the same time. It was originally conceptualised, just like AIDS, as a new kind of unidentified virus which burrows insidiously into your immune system and undermines it. People always talked about their immune systems collapsing. They bought supplements to boost their immune systems. You can probably still get them. It was incurable, controversial, political, terrifying and shameful. It had its activists, just like AIDS. And as soon as AIDS became containable, at least in the West, or treatable, and stopped being such a mystery, stopped being quite so fascinating an illness for doctors, and stopped being quite so scary to civilians, as soon as it stopped being in the news, stopped being so *political*, so ME as a diagnosis started to dwindle and disappear. People today feel just as tired, but they understand their situation differently. The politics of AIDS opened up the conceptual space, in which this idea of ME could thrive.'

Wow.

'Fascinating,' says Aly, who is slight and sharp and runs triathlons, has no arts degree, and is training to be an anaesthetist-traumatologist and will do well, I can tell. 'And how would you go about proving *that*?'

But something in what Klara says seems plausible to me. It is as if, for a while, ME was an acceptable way for people to be unwell – the symptoms, unwanted, congealing around them – and now it isn't. It was an epidemic that evolved and flourished in its ecological niche, and now, just as suddenly, is dwindling to extinction, and nobody seems to have any idea what it might have been.

It's not like this for all kinds of illness, of course. Illness, by and large, is as solid and real as the chair I'm sitting on: and nothing

I say or believe about it will change its nature. That's what people mean when they describe an illness as 'real'. You can see it and touch it, and if you can't do that, then at least you can measure it. You can weigh a tumour; you can see on the screen the ragged outline of the plaque of atheroma in your coronary artery which is occluded and crushing the life out of you, and you would be mad to question the *legitimacy* of this condition that prompts the wiry cardiologist to feed the catheter down the long forks and bends of your clogged arterial tree in order to feed an expanding metal stent into the blocked artery and save you.

No one questions the reality and medical legitimacy of those things in the world that can be seen, felt, weighed, touched. That creates a deep bias in the patient; it creates a profound preference among us, the healers.

But a person is *interactive*. Minds can't exist independently of other minds: that's the nature of our kind. The names we have for things in the world and the way that we choose to talk about them affect how we experience them. Our minds are made of language, and grammar, intentions, emotions, perceptions and memory. We can only experience the world through the agency of our minds, and how our minds interact with others. Science is a great tool for talking about the external world: the world that is indifferent to what *we* think. Science doesn't begin to touch the other, inner, social stuff. And that's a challenge in medicine. You need other tools for that.

'Shit-life syndrome,' offers Becky, whose skin is so pale it looks translucent, who wears white blouses with little ruffs buttoned to the top and her blonde hair in plaits, whose voice is vicarage English and in whose mouth *shit life* sounds anomalous. Medicine can have this coarsening effect. 'Shit-life syndrome provides the raw material. We doctors do all the rest.'

'Go on...'

'That's all I ever seem to see in GP. People whose lives are non-specifically crap. Women single parenting too many children, doing three jobs which they hate, with kids on Ritalin, heads wrecked by smartphone and tablet parenting. Women who hate their bodies and have a new diagnosis of diabetes because they're too fat. No wonder they want a better diagnosis! What am *I* meant to do?'

I like to keep this tutorial upbeat. I don't like it to become a moan-fest, which is pointless and damaging. Yet, I don't want to censor.

'... Sometimes I feel like a big stone, dropped into a river of pain. I create a few eddies around me, the odd wave or ripple, but the torrent just goes on...'

'... I see it different. It's worse! I think half the time we actually *cause* the problems. Or at least we create our own little side channels in the torrent. Build dams. Deep pools of misery of our own creation!'

That's Nadja. She's my trainee. And I recognise something familiar in what she is saying – the echo of something that I have said to her. It's flattering, and depressing.

'For example, take the issuing of sick notes. They're the worst. We have all of these people who say they're depressed, or addicted, or stressed, who stay awake all night because they can't sleep for worry, and sleep all day so they can't work, and they say they're depressed or anxious, or have backache or work-related stress, and we drug them up and sign them off, but what they're really suffering from are the symptoms of chronic unemployment and the misery of poverty, which are the worst illnesses that there are! And every time I sign one of these sick notes, I feel another little flake chipped off my integrity. You're asking about vectors for social illness? Sick notes! It's like we're ... shitting in the river, and worrying about the cholera!'

Strong words. I need to speak to Nadja about her intemperate opinions...

'At least, that's what *he* keeps saying,' says Nadja, nodding at me.

Nadja's father was a Croatian doctor, who fled the war there. Brought up as she was, at her father's knee, on his stories of war and torture, of driving his motorbike between Kiseljac and Sarajevo and all the villages in between with his medical bag perched on the back to do his house calls, she can never quite believe the sorts of things that pass for 'suffering' here. It doesn't make Nadja a more compassionate doctor. She sips her coffee, with a smile.

Aly, the one training to be an anaesthetist-traumatologist, says, 'We shouldn't do it. Simple as that. It's just not medicine. We should confine ourselves to the physical, and send the rest to a social worker, or a counsellor or a priest. No more sick notes, no more doing the dirty work of governments. If society has a problem with unemployment, that's society's problem, not mine. No more convincing people that they're sick. No more prescriptions for crap drugs that don't work. If you can't see it or measure it, it isn't real. We're *encouraging* all this pseudo-illness with our sick notes and our crap drugs. What's our first duty? *Do no harm!* End of.'

She'll be a great trauma doctor, no doubt about it.

'Can you think of any more concrete examples, in your experience, of doctors creating epidemics of new illnesses?'

I expect silence. The question is too hard.

'I can,' says Aly, after a moment.

I have contributed to this kind of harm myself. I must have. I have more than done my bit.

Skip back 20 years.

'Peter, do you remember that patient you saw just before you went away on holiday?'

I'm just back from Spain. Refreshed. Sun-drenched. Ready to begin the day. The world comes crashing back in. Angela, my partner in practice back then, looks at me with just that blend of concern, worry, and irritation which I had come to recognise. We are halfway between the coffee room and the patients' waiting room, a kind of quiet, semi-formal spot. It's not quite the ominous knock on the door, but neither is it a throwaway conversation in a public place.

'Jemma something,' says Angela.

I think *Borderas*. I think of her elf-like, sallow, washed-out look. The not-so-clean t-shirt, the black, henna-streaked hair. She had given me this odd look as she left my consulting room the last time I saw her, which I couldn't properly interpret.

Worry, perhaps. She was sceptical of my diagnosis. I had told her that she seemed depressed, but we both knew that I was stretching for some kind of legitimacy: a label we neither of us really believed. She had shrugged her shoulders as she left: the gesture said *yeah, whatever...*

Or betrayal? Perhaps that was it. That was what her look was saying: *I came to you, you let me down...*

And now I'm thinking *suicide?*

'Jemma Borderas,' I say holding it together. 'I thought that she was depressed. Prescribed her some…'

'I've seen her a couple of times. She was admitted to hospital. She's had what looks like a psychotic episode. Her flatmate found her trying to hang herself with a belt from her bedroom door. Apparently she's been cutting for ages. Anyway, she totally trashed her place and set off a fire alarm. They kept her in for a couple of days, but let her out on antipsychotics. She seems much better, but wants to see you again. Did you know she was cutting? Maybe you need to let the medical school know?'

I didn't know she was cutting, no. You see, I never asked her.

Same old Jemma comes in, just worse. I *see* the long sleeves now, the way she picks at her cuticles, pulls down the margins of her sleeves to cover her wrists. I notice the charcoal on her finger-tips, the bruises on her neck under her ears, both sides. She sits in agitated silence.

'What happened then Jemma?'

'Just freaked out.'

She sits in burning silence, stares at the floor, picks her nails.

'They're such a bunch of *fucking wankers!*'

'Who are?'

'*Medics!* The whole lot of them!' Unexpectedly, she smiles. Gives me this knowing smile from under her dark eyebrows.

Studying medicine can be like an initiation. For some the process of assimilation is frictionless, for others, it's a grind. I remember it. That's what she means by *medics!*

The smile has transformed her.

'But I'm fine now. I'll be okay.'

'How are you getting on with the antipsychotics?'

She stops smiling. Shakes her head. 'Didn't take them.'

'Why?'

'Make you fat. I looked it up in the BNF. Risperidone is for schizophrenia and psychosis, and they make you fat. I don't need them.'

'I think you might...'

'I just freaked out. Hadn't slept, had a drink or two, took a tab, on top of the ones you gave me. Just melted my brains. Can we not just leave it at that?'

Just melted my brains ... Not a legitimate diagnosis either.

'Not really. Having a ... psychotic episode. It has implications. For your training. We need to think about what we say to the medical school. Have you told them anything?'

She shakes her head, mouth like a clipped purse. 'I'm not ... *psychotic*...'

'But we still have to tell them.'

She shakes her head again. '*We?*'

I let it go. Pause a moment.

'I understand that you've been ... cutting?'

'That's just something that I do. It's nothing. It got bad. Now it's under control.'

'Show me?'

She raises her sleeves. Tiny weals, reaching from cuff line to the margin of her raised sleeve. Some white, old and flat, spiderwebs of old scars, some still pink and healing, a few fresh steri-strips on her wrists from the other night. The years of pain, and the release from pain, written like that on her body. I want to gasp. I suppress the urge to gasp. I'm not her mum.

'What do you use?'

'Scalpel.'

'Every day?'

'Mostly.'

'Do you want help with that?'

'No.' Unequivocally. 'It's my thing. *Everyone* at medical school does it. Where *I* go you're either a cutter, a chucker or a starver, and I like my food. It's under control. It *helps.*'

I start to frame my next question: *Why? What happened to you? What about the scars? How can you do this …? Stop it!* But no question makes sense in the face of her unequivocal 'No.' Her apparent indifference. Besides, as she says, all the girls do it.

'How did you get on with Jemma Borderas?' asks Angela, later on, as she kindly makes me tea.

We doctors screw up all the time. Good doctors understanding this are kind to one another. Only the lousy ones condemn. Choose your colleagues with care. Angela looked out for me.

'Badly. She really got away from me, Jemma.'

———————

'Cyclical Vomiting Syndrome with Abdominal Pain,' says Aly.

'What's that?'

'It's a common, geographically and temporally localised condition, which is found in the A&E department of the Queen Elizabeth Hospital, Inverteuchter, on every other Tuesday and every other weekend.'

?

'Seriously.'

Everyone is laughing, everyone thinks that Aly is joking, other than Rebecca, who obviously knows something that the rest of us don't.

'Everyone knows about it! There's this consultant, Dr Mcrudden – he's a really really lovely physician. Everyone wants to be his patient, he's lovely to the juniors, everyone wants to work with him, apart from the nurses, who all think that he's crap. He gets all the fibromyalgia and irritable bowel syndrome patients. So, Dr Mcrudden has this cohort of people who present to casualty every time he's the consultant on duty. They turn up with vomiting and abdominal pain, and they get treated with morphine and antiemetics, and then they go home. They have a special named patient protocol for them and everything. Whenever one of them comes in, it's morphine 10mg IV and 50mg of cyclizine. We just turn them around as fast as possible. The problem is some of the other consultants will have nothing to do with it. They all think there's no such diagnosis. They think it's not *real*. So the patients have a Facebook page. I've seen it – it's like one of these angry-patient support groups you get. So every morning one or other of them turns up at A&E first thing, finds out if it's one of the *sympathetic* consultants on duty,' indicating 'sympathetic' in air-quotes, 'and then posts it on Facebook, and then the rest all come along. It's a real pain. It's becoming a real problem. It would be easier if they just posted the consultant rota at the front door, maybe put a little hypodermic logo next to the "nice" ones.'

'That's … shocking.'

'But they're all morphine addicts, yeah?'

'No … that's the thing. They're not. It would be easy if they were. They sort of seamlessly graduate from other illnesses. Some *are* like proper addicts, but most aren't. There are students, and nurses, and manual workers, secretaries, bus drivers, lots of care workers. They're all sorts. They've even got some children with it. But they're all, all of them, absolutely convinced that they've got this thing "Cyclical Vomiting with Abdominal Pain Syndrome", CVAPS, and they need their treatment. I've seen them. They're not faking it. They're really in pain. Or they think they are. But only on alternate Tuesdays, and alternate weekends.'

'*Really?*'
'Really.'

Jemma would always say that it's 'her thing' when I asked, then turn the conversation to something else.

I hadn't thought at first that we had made much of a connection, she and I, but something grew between us: she kept coming back to see me. She would sit, answer my concern with monosyllables, look at the carpet, and from time to time reward me with her smile. She would roll up her sleeve when I insisted, and show to me the lace-work pattern of tiny scars on her arms, the new and the old, and if I pushed her she would say again, 'It helps! Everyone does it! You wouldn't hassle me if it was just a tattoo, would you?'

No. Probably not. A doctor with different, better skills, might have found a way for her to talk. Perhaps there was something there to be interpreted, some fact that was *true*, an explanation that would be helpful, for why Jemma cut, but if there was, I never found it, and when I tried to ask, she would roll her eyes, or smile, or look at the floor, and say, 'It's just my thing', or 'Everyone does it'.

I didn't tell the medical school about her psychotic episode. I'm quite sure that I should have, obviously – there were rules – but the time was never quite right, and then the moment had passed.

She dropped out for a year, against my advice, planning to go travelling, and 'get her head together', and I thought *That's it, she'll be gone. She won't come back.* But she did, to my surprise, and she came to see me at the start of her final year. And, as happens, when she came back, she had changed. Her hair had grown in its natural colour, and she had decluttered her piercings. She was starting to look more like a doctor. She had spent a year working in her uncle's garage in Girona, made a little money, then travelled. Her scars, by then, were almost all old. A person who didn't know, might not even notice.

I left that practice. I needed to move on. During my last couple of weeks, pleasingly, many of my patients came to see me just to say farewell. There were many surprises. Jemma was one of them.

'I wanted to say goodbye,' said the new, adult, Jemma. 'You really, really helped me.'

As is so often the case, *I didn't do a thing*. Nonetheless, there is a smirr of tears. I blink them away.

'Thank you. You look like you're going to make it through.'

'Amazing, eh? Things are going okay now. I should get through.'

'What do you plan to do?'

'Gonna be a GP, I think. Or mebbe a shrink.' She laughs at the irony, smiling her old smile.

'You'll be good at it.'

'I brought you something.' She is carrying a long, unwieldy package. 'Open it.'

———

Yvette: 'Cutting. Surely *that's* got to be new!'

For as long as there are people with limbs and blades, I think, *they will cut.* I glance at my picture on the wall, and hear Jemma's voice saying 'Cutters, chuckers or starvers…' and think *Are they still?* Or is that an epidemic that came and went? I look at the six trainees. I'm scarcely talking now. When a tutorial goes well, I do no work. I lob in a few ideas, and they run with them. They are smart, clean, well informed, always do their homework, always bring their stethoscopes. A little complacent maybe, sometimes prone to judge, but they'll be fine. They're not 'cutters, chuckers or starvers'. They don't 'melt their brains'.

'All the mad slashers!' says Yvette, chatty. 'The self-harmers: the slicers, burners, pill-takers, wall-punchers. They're the ones that *I* can't handle! Every night in A&E, it's like a pain factory, and they all come in, pissed and angry, especially when I'm on duty. And I'm so tired! Yet I'm still meant to be *nice* to them! And they're so *manipulative!* You try to be kind, they just come back, and if you're horrid to them, they just cut again to spite you, and then complain!'

Yvette is the angriest. She contributes least, and so I never know what she's thinking. She's the only one about whom I have any doubts. The one who, when she moans, isn't just letting off steam, but *really* seems to mean it. There's pain powering Yvette's tirades. She means to train as a physician. I sort of hope not to become too ill when she's on duty.

'I mean, how did we get like this? How did it become so that cutting became such a common, *accepted* means of self-expression? Has it *always* been like this?'

'My little sister cuts...,' says Aly, and the room goes suddenly quiet.

That's how it happens. You create a safe place, where people can share what they *really* think, or what they *think* they really think, and what they *really think* can be quite uncomfortable. An energy is created: people are carried in this flood of angry, judgy, unconsidered, unacceptable words, and then some quiet voice says something like 'My little sister cuts' and the temperature in the room goes down. Everyone goes quiet.

I think that's good. The jeopardy is high. The emotions are real. It's how people learn.

Yvette immediately goes pale. Yvette shuts up. Yvette feels terrible. Yvette has learned something important.

'She's still at school,' says Aly. 'She's quite a few years behind me. She's the bright one – always straight As, *and* she plays the viola.' She smiles a watery smile, and the others in the room make way to let her speak.

'She always had a bit of an eating thing, but we all ignored it because we all thought she was doing fine. But in her A-level year, she just got really, really anxious. She didn't know whether to go to medical school like me, or to go to a conservatoire to study viola. She got really crazy obsessed with it, just working and practising 20 hours a day, not sleeping, not eating. She had counselling and stuff, and was on antidepressants, but she just seemed to get worse. She was working *all the time*, and getting full marks, but she still wasn't happy. Anyway…'

The room stays quiet.

'… Anyway … we were on holiday, in Italy and it was *roasting* hot. We were going swimming, and Pippa always liked swimming but she wouldn't take her stuff off. She kept on going around in these stupid long trousers and long sleeves. My mum and dad didn't even notice. I think they were just in denial, but I kind of confronted her…'

The room stays quiet.

'… she'd been doing it for *ages*.' Quite suddenly Aly is weeping. Aly's tears are shocking.

We all have in our minds this same image: the same image that is in hers. A swimming pool, Tuscan hills, the sun, the blue-green

cypress trees, the stick thin girl, baring her arms, her legs, the
pink lines, the purple lines, the etchings of pain. Aly weeps.

'Nobody knew.'

———

'I have a theory,' I announce, a month later, the next time we all
meet. 'It might help.'

Two pairs of eyes swivel to meet mine. Two dip below the
margins of their clasped hands to engage with screens. *Not a bad
ratio*, I think. Together, Yvette and Aly are making tea.

'It's this. The ways that we feel ourselves to be unwell, and
the way that we behave when we are unwell, depend on available social and medical models of illness and behaviour. But we
have this compelling sense, this *illusion* of an executive self who
commands the physical actions and behaviours of our body, and
feels sensations that arise from the external world. If there were
fakery to be done in the performance of illness, that *self* would
be the culprit. It's the agent we all sense inside. It makes the idea
that behaviours can *evolve* feel too passive to be plausible. But
there is evidence that it doesn't work like that. Has anyone heard
of a Canadian neurophysiologist called Benjamin Libbet?'

Klara makes to answer. I cut across her.

'Libbet conducted experiments on the brains of volunteers,
relating intention to action. He showed, using real time PET
scanning, that the conscious intention to conduct a simple
act, moving a subject's arm, or formulating a sentence, took
place *after* the physical initiation of movement. It suggests that
conscious intention has no direct causal relationship with physical action and behaviour. Game changing, eh?'

One of the two remaining pairs of eyes dips down to a screen.
Aly and Yvette interrupt with tea and scones.

'Intention and behaviour are aspects of the same thing. They evolve together.'

With Jemma watching still, I unwrap her gift.

A vertical triptych: three views of a mountain. The top, in oil, thickly applied, all reds and blacks, storm-clouds gathered on a summit. The second, a watercolour, a spring day, the sense of a breeze cutting the surface of the water at the base of a volcano capped with snow, a scattering of ships by the shore. Her name, signed in pencil in the corner, almost invisible: *Jemma Borderas*. The third, a single sweep of a calligraphy brush, a steep up-and-down stroke, a cupped summit, and a symbol, a Japanese character at its side. *Sympathy*. Or *Peace*. Or *Friendship*. *The Passing of Time*. Something like that.

Opiates are the Opiate
of the People: Part 1

'You never *listen*!' says Gale, punchy as always, more irritated than usual. 'I bet *you've* never had a heroin problem! I bet you've never had to *just say no*!'

Twice offered actually, but both times declined. The second time regretted, perhaps.

When I was a student, I spent a time travelling and working in Northern Pakistan.

That period, the elective term, was at least notionally educational, and for the more serious students it was. The ones that really cared organised for themselves three months experience in cardiac surgery, or anaesthetics, or neurology, and these were the ones that all seemed to get the best jobs in their chosen subjects when they qualified. These were the ones that really flew. Others of us, who struggled more to get airborne, saw it as a kind of study holiday with benefits, and back then when life was kinder and easier for middle-class white boys like me to sort of rattle through life as we pleased and only needed to turn up from time to time, it was an opportunity to loosen ourselves of the shackles of study, kick back, and travel. It was a time for the most perfect freedom.

My friend Andy had recently returned from a mountaineering trip to the Karakorum, where he had climbed to over 6000 metres on Mushtaq Tower and come back changed entirely — lean and fit, with a seared look to the skin and a far-off gaze in the eye which is rare in men who come from Fife. On a big screen in my brother's flat in Edinburgh, he showed us photos of dragon-teeth peaks and dazzling white ice fields and men in glacier glasses, men draped in the ironmongery of serious climbing, and men drinking tea and puffing on a hookah on the veranda of a wooden government guest house by a deep grey river in a town called Ashkole. We sat around drinking beer; it was dark outside and raining, and I thought *I want some of that*. I have always revered Andy for all sorts of reasons.

The expedition doctor, a GP from Anstruther, kindly gave me the address for the military hospital in Skardu. He had spent a little time there, met a chap called Ali Mustafa, the duty surgeon, who had drained an abscess for him. He felt sure that Ali would welcome a medical student. I felt sure that he would too and wrote to him, a polite letter in my clearest English on flimsy blue airmail paper saying how much I wanted to study surgery in the Northern Karakorum, and a month or two later, received a reply on a post card, written in smudged red crayon, indicating, or so I thought, that I might come. The card had obviously been a long time in transit and was somewhat water damaged, but it seemed good enough to me, and good enough for my director of studies in

Manchester when I presented it to him, saying that I was off to study surgery *in Pakistan*!

I wasn't expected.

Of course I wasn't expected. My post card with its scarcely legible red squiggle was worthless. There was no Dr Ali Mustafa now. There had been, but he was long gone: had left under something of a cloud too, or so it seemed, though people in Skardu were too polite to say, thinking that he must somehow be my friend.

Major Sammi Ulah Khan sat in his office in pressed immaculate tan-coloured Major's uniform and looked at me through his pale blue eyes. He was flanked by two unranked, bearded men, one with henna adorning his thick black hair, both in sharply creased fatigues. There were post-surgical patients in dressings lying on charpoys in the corridor outside. There were flies everywhere and the place had a thick, ripe, sweet smell, like rotting apples. Skardu military hospital was the drop point for casualties from a slow burn conflict with India, occurring on the frontier glacier, about 20 miles away. Men were taken to the front on the open backs of jeeps: poor boys from Sind and the Punjab, where it is *really hot*, who had no equipment for glacier fighting.

Major Sammi looked tired. His hospital was full of amputations, frost bite, and bullet wounds. I had travelled for six days by train and rickshaw up the length of the Indus and the Karakoram Highway and was ragged and smelt bad. But *no one* in Pakistan smelt bad. If your job in Pakistan was to sluice out the polo ponies' stables after your evening shift in the rendering plant, you still finished the day smelling of primroses.

Major Sammi looked through tired pale blue eyes at the 20-year-old with his crappy red beard and incipient dysentery. Somewhere from the mountains came the far-off drone of a helicopter and Major Sammi seemed suddenly to waken.

'Of course you are welcome, Dr Dorward,' he said, in heavily accented yet still cultured English. 'You may stay for as long as you wish. You may reside in the doctors' mess.' He glanced at the door, and his two men jumped to lead me away. Major Sammi twice tapped a thick sheaf of paper on his desk in the decisive manner of busy people in 1985, and reached for his cap from the hat-stand. The drone of approaching helicopters grew louder.

I think I owe a lifetime's debt to the people of Pakistan. It happened to me, over and over again, for three months. I would end up somewhere, destitute and hungry, at the mercy of strangers and a total pain in the arse, and then I would be fed, and given a bed.

A year or two later, just after knocking off a three-day wall-to-wall shift as a junior obstetrician in St Mary's in Manchester, I was stopped on the pavement outside the hospital by a totally lost, shambly guy in his early thirties dressed in shalwar kameez and a chapati cap, who asked me in appallingly accented English, 'Too much lost – where, Sir, is this?' and thrust under my nose a handwritten address somewhere in Droylsden, which was miles away. I said to him 'Wait!' which he didn't understand, so I tried again with forefinger raised for emphasis and said 'wait!' and he seemed to get it, because when I dashed off to get my car which was parked in the basement car-park and got back he was still there, bewildered with his scrap of paper, so I picked him up and drove him to Droylsden where his anxious family were waiting for him. They must have thought that I was a taxi. So somewhere from Pakistan I absorbed something, for a while: some alien spirit or essence of the place, of obligation, or generosity.

Memory postcards from Pakistan:

+ A dimly lit operating theatre. Flies. That smell again, of rotting fruit. Through a cracked window, a view across to an orchard of apricot trees. A child with peritonitis on the table with her abdomen open, but it's all far too late.
+ My day off, and I walk five miles into the hills, to Satpara Lake, where I swim in cold glacier water. I pass an intricate Buddhist rock carving on the way, set well back from the road, edges worn flat by age and human touch, a well-beaten track still leading to it. At the lake, a boy of 12 or so comes and sits beside me: there is something he wants to communicate with me, urgently, and I don't understand what it is that he is trying to say. I realise later that he was trying to sell me sex.
+ A postcard of mountains. Guts churning. Starving. Nausea, and breathless in the thin air. Climbing the shoulder of the hill above the hospital to try to get that view across the Indus valley to the high Karakorum and realising too late that this walk would take me days. Dispirited, I return in darkness, loneliness carving out its hollow in my chest.
+ Sitting at the end of the day having tea outside a tea-shack by the road. Low sun filters through wood-smoke. Two young men pass by, hand in hand, one wears a garland of yellow flowers in his hair. The smell of stables – polo ponies – and kerosene. A first deep inhalation, K2 cigarettes! and a bubble of contentment swelling.

+ Walking in the narrow streets of old Peshawar. Today is Ashura, the Shia day of mourning, but I don't know that. There are crowds of men in the streets. They grow dense and hostile; there is a tension in the air which I haven't experienced before, and I'm fearful and try to escape, but can't. I am locked in, in a flow of men, trapped in a dusty little square ringed by tall, old buildings with wooden grills overlooking the street. Men are beating their chests; men are beating their backs with chains swung from short wooden handles. There are chains, knives and ring-pulls. They cut deeply; there is a frenzy of sweat and blood. Crowded in the shadows behind the wooden grills above are women: I know them by their voices. Their excitation, their crying and murmuring, calls and sobs, are like bird song.

+ Reading by paraffin light in the doctors' mess. It's cold outside, with the sun down, but warm here. We share tea and chat, and then they go off, altogether, elsewhere, to pray. I realise, months later, that I was occupying their prayer space. They don't ask me to leave; they don't want me to feel awkward.

+ Opium. A government guesthouse with a verandah, on the banks of the Shyok river. Grey meltwater tumbling from the high glaciers, boulders the size of cars rolling and bouncing down the valley floor. I spend a week in Khapalu with a man who becomes a friend, and the Emir of Khapalu organises a lift for me back to Skardu with a group of five young Afghan men – farmers, smugglers, soldiers, I don't know, because we don't share any words. In 20 years' time this kind of relationship would be impossible, but right now they treat me well: somewhere between a distinguished foreign emissary, and a family pet. They like it when I perform tricks: juggling with three apricots, or reading aloud in English, from *Great Expectations*. They wear cloth turbans, and immaculate white shalwar kameez, and live out of little canvas shoulder bags with Russian letters on. They carry guns. In the evening after a day of travel they cook rice and oily paratha on a kerosene stove and drink tea as the sun goes down. We sit on the veranda. Slightly furtive, one unpacks his hookah, a wallet of thick brown paper enclosing a wad of brownish paste which melts, burns and bubbles in the bowl, and each sucks deeply on the nectar and leans back on his chair to witness the emerging stars. The youngest hesitates, then offers me the chewed mouthpiece.

In one version of this story I inhaled the cooled smoke deeply, swallowed its sourness and leant back contented and drowsy in my chair to search the turquoise sky for Tarek, the evening star. In another I raised my palm politely to decline, thanked them in the cool Presbyterian way, but … no.

'Are you listening to me, Doctor! *You've* never used it, so you just don't know, do you?'

'No … I … No…'

Gale, I confess it. I was miles away.

A young man in a turban and a black beard hawks and spits into the fire, smiles through the gaps in his teeth, draws on a hookah. The rumble of stones from the river below. The evening star, bright and low in the sky…

Sometimes when I'm at work I have these *epic* daydreams.

'So you can't really *say*, can you? Don't get me wrong, you seem like a nice enough wee fellow, Doctor, but every time I come here I get *this*…' She makes a yapping on gesture with her right hand in the air between our two faces – *yap yap yap* – and continues, 'but really, with all due respect, etc., you have to acknowledge when you admonish me to, what was it, to stop using heroin, *stop jagging*! Yer kinda speaking through a hole in your, well, you know what…'

A bit of context: Gale uses words like 'acknowledge' and 'admonish', which is unusual. She's in her mid-forties. She has intelligent, sparkly eyes and a nice smile, which is hard-won. Scrubbed up and with some serious wardrobe and dental work, Gale might plausibly sit on my side of the desk. She said once, 'What you have to understand, Doctor, is that most junkies are as thick as shit, but I'm not.' She also told me: 'You know the best thing I've ever done? Not having children. If you have children, you get a flat and you get benefits, and you can get out of this shit. But I wouldn't do that to a child. I said I wasn't going to bring a child into *this* world, and I didn't. That absent child? Best thing *I've* never done!'

She is articulate, clever, forceful, foul, likeable, and broken. Her dog had diabetes and was taken away from her and destroyed because she so neglected him. She grieved and grieved for that dog. Today she has an abscess in her groin, discharging thick, blood-streaked pus. She showed it to me behind the curtain, squeezed it a little while I got a swab, and said bleakly, half laughing, '*Yeuch*, that's *minging!*' in a tone of voice which, I don't know why, enraged me, broke my heart. It prompted me to say that thing I oughtn't: 'You just *have to* … stop … *jagging!*' which is what really got her going.

'What the *fuck* gives you the right to tell me? With your ... head full of teeth and your lovely kids? You don't *know*! Lecturing doesn't help. Do you think I don't know it all already?'

'So what *should* I do?'

'Just ... do your job and be helpful. Stop judging! Listen! People like me, we judge ourselves enough already!'

Okay. Pause. Try to rescue this.

'I'll give you antibiotics for your groin. Tell me if it isn't getting better, and I'll arrange to have it drained. Now tell me. What else can I say or do that would be helpful?'

She looks at her shoes. Broken plastic trainers. She clasps her hands. The rest of her is fine boned, but her hands are swollen and puffy: she has injected for so long that the fine blood vessels in her hands are destroyed, her feet as well. Scrub up, fix her teeth and her clothes: changed and transformed though she might become, nothing will ever make that better: she'll always have these odd, puffy hands and feet.

She pauses. She says, 'You're always trying to change people. Do you think anyone *wants* to be like this? I've been a junkie for so long now that even thinking about not being a drug addict is painful. I don't even know if I want to think about it. And every time I've tried to stop, I've got all these new best pals chapping on my door, shouting "Come on Gale, one last wee burn!", and I always let them in.'

'Why?'

She looks at me as if I'm stupid.

'They'll just keep hammering on my door otherwise.'

'And they won't leave you alone?'

'As my Grandma used to say, "Every stottery cow needs a pal".'

What?

'It takes a village to grow a child. It takes a village to grow a junkie too. People like us are the only people we know!'

Gale never chose to be like this. To suggest that she might have just seems silly. *When, exactly, did you* choose *to be what you are?* Gale didn't choose her parents, nor did she choose to miss those few opportunities which arose for her in her school where too few of the teachers had the wit or the time to tell her apart from the crowd. Gale didn't choose whichever smoky-breathed man it was that climbed into her bed and did whatever it was that he did that set her on her way. (There's always a man. Someone like Gale may take long enough to tell you, but get to know her well, build that trust, and in the end she might. There's always a man at the beginning of the story.) Gale didn't choose that her father be violent. She didn't choose the bad set she fell in with when she was a child, nor did she choose the rain-hammered tenements where she has lived out her adulthood. She never chose to live in a world where what passes for heroin is passed from hand to hand in tiny cling-film 'burn bags', where what passes for the exotic, what once was opium, is flour and baking powder cut with codeine, which is burned on tinfoil and inhaled, or mixed in company with a squeeze of lemon juice, boiled on a spoon and injected, where it sits, bubbling under the skin, and ferments into the kind of smelly, discharging abscess which she brings for me to see, here, today.

She didn't *choose*. What happened to Gale, just happened, just the same as for any of us. No one chooses. Not really. In a world so determined, what could that possibly even mean: *to choose?*

I want to write about free will: about how, in a determined universe, the very idea of freedom makes no sense, because there is no place for it. I want to write about how free will is an illusion, and its consequences – blame, wickedness, responsibility, culpability – are illusions too. I want to make the case that, in such a world, there can be no place for punishment, for harming, restricting, incarcerating a person for the bad things that have happened to them. Things that never happened to the judge, nor to you or me. But when I think of Gale, my argument falls away. Because, illusion or not, Gale wants more than anything to be the kind of thing in the world that *chooses*, and chooses better. Gale yearns so much to be this kind of thing, a thing that can *make choices*, that even to think about it causes her pain. She had laughed bleak laughter, with a cold shower of tears, when she showed me her groin, and what she had done to it.

———————

Twice offered, both times declined.

The second time in Pakistan; the first time in a student union, in 1983, one evening, sitting on my own, nursing a half pint, not knowing a soul.

A posh chap in a blazer came and sat by me, started talking about his girlfriend, Sarah, whom it was established, by sheer coincidence, I had known at school. I took an instant, poisonous dislike to him. I don't know why. Men in their twenties shouldn't wear blazers.

He said, confidingly, after a while, 'I'm dreadfully fond of heroin,' looking at me with raised eyebrows as if to ask 'Are you?' I said no. Of course I said no. I loathed him. I walked away, left him to it.

Good choice, I think, though really, for me, no choice at all.

———————

The usual understanding is that it is the drug that enslaves. It is the drug that works the change on people. Get rid of the drug and you get rid of the problem.

My next patient this morning is Mikey. He's already ten minutes late for his appointment, but I know that whatever I say, I'll end up having to see him. So while we wait, imagine for a moment you are Mikey's mother. Remember when your child was a bonny bright tousle-haired wee thing that called you 'mummy' and knew, properly, how to love? Remember the time? The time you think of as *before?* Do you remember how, when he was 12 or 13, he fell in with a group of older boys? Your husband saw no harm in it, but you did. Although you gave him love and treats and sat him down and tried to get him to talk to you, you sensed that you were losing him, but didn't know why, and you didn't know what to do, because some devilry, some temptation, made him prefer them to you.

You remember, much later, that sense that something unknown was sucking the blood and vitality from him. How his skin grew pale and grey, almost translucent, his muscle turned to mush that you could almost see the fat and bones beneath. Hard times to recollect, but you must make yourself ask, obsessively, over and over, for a boy so loved, *how could it go so wrong?*

Do you remember that almost imperceptibly slow transition as he turned from the child you loved, your only boy, into that hungry grey ghost that stole money from your purse? Do you remember the week in Saltcoats at the caravan, when he was 14, when he seemed to get better for a bit, when he ran along the beach with his dog, throwing sticks, and you thought *I've been imagining it — he's fine! I've been imagining it all?* Do you remember how long you spent turning a blind eye to the money that was missing from your bank accounts? Sometimes in the dark of the night you make a reckoning. Twenty years have passed and now he's 32. Leaving aside the squandered love, the emotional pain and the broken marriage, how much has he cost you? You think about the thefts, the debts paid, the jewellery pawned and lost forever, and tot it up, hating yourself as you do. The money that he stole from your friends, that you made good. You try not to think too much about that one, but at night you can't not, because the thought comes to you from out of the dark of its own accord.

The damage to the front door when it was kicked in by the police. The costs associated with the law. The taxi fares to and from court. Covering up absences from work with fake illnesses. This bitter accounting is *your* private addiction. The car you bought, then had to sell. The endless, unpayable loans, and the cleaning job you've taken on at night to pay off the interest. Sometimes at night, on your own, you make a reckoning. If you're honest, you think, it's about 70K. Give or take.

You have this fantasy that he will be returned to you one day, healed and free of drugs, a little older perhaps, perhaps a little battered, but *free* and you feel your heart leaping up like a dog, hungry for affection, hungry for the hand that proffers this dream, this cruel dream. You also have a fantasy that he is dead.

At night, it's this second that calms you.

The folk understanding holds that it is the drug that makes you its slave. On the face of it, that makes a lot of sense. A generation of psychological experimentation dating back to the sixties seems to have proven it. If you place laboratory rats in Skinner boxes (cages, measuring 7" by 8" arranged in banks), provide each indi-vidual rat with food, water and free access to morphine, your rat will preferentially feed on morphine and neglect the rest. The rat will neglect everything, in fact, until it is too weak to reach the teat on the bottle with opiate – at which point it will die. Some resist; some are resistant to the allure of the drug, and continue to thrive, insofar as thriving is possible, but the vast majority don't. The dice are loaded against you if you are a rat in a Skinner box with access to morphine. That's the argument for legal prohibition: get rid of the morphine in the cage and your rats do fine. The model seems to work well, for rats. It's extraordinary how quickly, how *easily*, it has been generalised to people.

They start off as diverse as everyone else that we know, but for people who fall to using street heroin quite quickly it works its thing, quite quickly you start conforming to a kind. Like the rats in their cages, your skin goes grey, your teeth rot in their gums, your coat, your hair, your clothes are dirty and you stop looking after yourself. You become *antisocial*. You adopt the junkie voice – a kind of gravelly whine, a querulous beseeching that is enraging and intolerable to be around – and you are constantly, crudely, wheedling and manipulative, in order to obtain not just drugs, but any kind of trivial advantage at all. That's the worst: you are sick, as sick as it's possible to be. But kindness doesn't seem to work in the usual way: it seems to make things worse. The kinder I am to you, the more you use me. The more of myself that I offer you, the harder I am betrayed. I feel used. There is nothing worse than being *used*.

The model is beguiling. How quickly, how easily people can seem to conform to it, like rats locked in their cages.

Mikey's turned up for his appointment at long last.

'My mum says that this is my last chance. She says that if I let her down again, then I'm out.'

I check his date of birth and do a kind of double-take. He's *32*! With his baseball cap and his half hoisted jeans showing his grubby Bawbags boxers, he looks like a teenager. He's even been brought along by his mum, who's a patient of mine as well. A respectable, well-kept woman, dogged by the shame of it, she has tried *so hard* for the boy – she works as a receptionist in a car wash during the day, and has a cleaning job at night. There's a kind of low-level gangster in my neck of the woods that scents out the boys whose mothers love them still, like sharks scent blood. You bleed the child, then you bleed the mother: it's an income stream that's good for years. Mikey's mum has just sold her house and is moving out, into a caravan. You can almost smell the blood in the water.

Despite the many harsh words that have passed between us, I quite like Mikey. Hidden deep, imperceptible to most, he has some of his mother's kindness, her intelligence. Though not today. He stares up at me through wide open, imploring eyes.

'So I'm back, Doctor. You've just *got* to help me.'

There's a gleam of sweat on his grey skin. He's shaking. His mouth smells like a blocked drain in summer. The spiderweb tattoo on his neck is livid and sharp. He looks like shit. Mikey had been on a prescription for 30ml of methadone, which isn't a lot, for a couple of years, and had been doing okay. He had a job in the car wash for a bit, but lost it, because they found out that he was on methadone, and then he'd stopped picking up his prescription, which is always a bad sign.

'It's snakes and ladders, Doctor,' which is something that relapsed heroin addicts say. 'But this is it, if I carry on like this, if ah dinnae stop jagging, I'm deid. Ah've got tae clean up. Besides,' he says, solemnly, 'I've got the bairn now. It's a new start.'

The bairn?

'Aye, did you no ken? I've got a grandchild now. Last Tuesday. My daughter says I cannae see her unless I clean up…'

Daughter? Granddaughter?

One of the paradoxes of heroin addiction is how oddly it ages you. Mikey's lungs are the lungs of a heavy-smoking 60-year-old. Every morning he coughs green pus, his tubes having filled with phlegm; he has chronic obstructive pulmonary disease. He also has coronary artery disease, though we don't know it yet, and in 10 years' time he will have angina, or heart failure, or be dead. He has liver cirrhosis from hepatitis C, and he walks with a stick. His skin is finely lined and thin, like a 60-year-old, and his skin hangs from his belly like a man who once had muscle or fat, and has lost it.

Mikey is frightened that his mother will be angry with him and throw him out of the house. Mikey is prone to stealing and to having tantrums. Mikey has no bank account of his own. Mikey whines and wheedles and lies around all day playing on his computer. Mikey is a lost 15-year-old, locked in time, locked in the body of a dying old man.

'So how are you going to clean up?'

He looks at his trainers. Looks up at me.

'I can't believe that I'm saying this again…'

A tear of self-pity.

'I know I've let you down, Doctor, and I'm sorry. I've let my mum down too. I've let my daughter down. I've even let *myself* down…'

One aspect of Mikey's unlovable childishness is his habit of trying to make everyone else around him into his mum.

So get to the point Mikey.

'I'd like another prescription for methadone. Please.'
I pause. I nod. *Okay.*
'Here's how it works…'

Here's how it works. It's about harm reduction: palliation, not cure. There is no cure.

Mikey will get no prescription today. Mikey will have to step over a series of tiny, tiny hurdles before he gets his methadone. Call this paternalistic? This *is* paternalistic. Mikey will have to chew on a wad of absorbent cellulose, a kind of dry swab, so that I can collect his saliva to determine what he is *actually* taking. Removing the deceit creates the possibility of truth telling, opens a space in which an honest conversation can happen. Nothing enslaves like lies: both deceiver and deceived. I stopped taking urine samples a while ago: too many faked tests, too many bottles of children's urine, spiked with methadone – a cold, greenish sample. That's *why* they make methadone green.

Baby steps to adulthood.

Mikey will be required to never miss appointments, to never be late, and to turn up at the chemist every day to be given his methadone, under supervision, to ensure that he isn't selling it on to those other grey wraiths that haunt the chemist's door on methadone days.

Mikey will be required to come back to see me in a few days, on time, having had no opiates for 24 hours, so that I can see that he is withdrawing: I don't want to create an opiate habit where there was none before, although in Mikey's case, this seems quite unlikely.

I will see Mikey every week, step up his methadone in slow increments, 5 to 10ml at a time, until he eventually hands me spit samples that are free of drugs. He will start to look better. He will wash, get his teeth fixed, lose that maddening, wheedling tone he adopts when things are bad. He will start to be ... *honest*.

Baby steps to adulthood.

I will space out his appointments, space out his visits to the chemist, dispense him a little more trust, as if trust is the potency that heals him. Perhaps in time he will get a job, come off benefits, have a little money to buy things for his granddaughter. Perhaps his daughter, in time, will let her father see her child.

After a few long years, Mikey will come to see me, or my successor, and say, 'By the way, Doc, I came off the methadone.' And I or my successor will raise an eyebrow, and he will say, 'Aye, I just looked at myself in the mirror, and I said, fuck it, 52 years old ... I stopped about four months ago, and I've not looked back.'

'Was it a struggle?'

'Nah. It was the bairn really, she just looked at me one day and she says "why are you still *on* that shite grandpa?" She's off to college next year! She wants to be a nurse...'

It happens. Every year, I see it, once or twice, maybe.

Mikey will have grown up. And the ghost of his dead mother will be singing and dancing among the clouds.

But today there is a snag. He comes back to see me five days later, bang on the appointed time. He is pale and shaky. His pupils are dilated and he looks like he has a fever. He is antsy, tamping down his own irritation, mustering all the niceness he can find so that nothing can stop me from giving him the methadone that he needs. He has clearly had no opiates for the 24 hours that we agreed. He's kept up his side of the deal. He looks at me impatiently, tamping down his impatience.

'There's a snag...'

His face says *Oh, fuck...*

'What...?'

'The sample you gave me ... it *was* yours, wasn't it?'

'You saw me chewing it. You put it in the bag. Is there a problem?'

I've seen this before. I've encountered this problem before. This problem is far commoner than you might think.

'There wasn't any heroin in the spit sample.'

'But that's not ... I've been using every day for *weeks* ... There's something wrong with the test...'

'There was some codeine, some gabapentin, some tramadol, but no heroin.'

'... right...'

'So that crap you buy from the friend, whatever, who sells you what you think is heroin?'

The penny is...

'He's not your friend. It might be all kind of crap you're smoking, but it's not heroin.'

... the penny finally drops.

'Fuck.'

The withdrawals are imagined? But he still has gooseflesh. His heart is racing, he is sweaty, he shakes, his pupils are dilated, his nostrils flare like a trapped animal's. But they are imagined.

Pause.

'So will you still give me my methadone, Doctor?'

So it's not the substance that is the problem. Not *just* the substance.

Listen to Gale. That's what she keeps on saying to me:

'Can you not *listen* to what I'm trying to tell you, Doctor? It's not people that use drugs, it's communities! Do you drink alcohol? With your doctor friends?'

I don't respond to this one – never do – it's unprofessional.

'*All* drug use is cultural.'

From time to time, in different cities, in different countries, the state is successful in the war it wages against those people that buy and sell the substances it deems illegal. For a time at least, the amount of heroin in the stuff that's sold as 'heroin' drops to zero, near enough. In Toronto, in the nineties, the police, by a fluke, intercepted *all* the heroin being imported by a monopoly supplier, and for many months there was an absolute heroin drought. The effect on the city's drug trade was remarkably small. Traders still bought and sold small wraps of what they called 'heroin'. Their clients still got together in groups and cooked it up and smoked or injected it. It still burned holes in their lungs, and fizzed and fermented under their skin, and they still experienced something of what it was they sought to experience, and they still withdrew from the drug when they couldn't access it. The odd cohesive *culture* of heroin use continues, even in the absence of heroin.

Listen to Gale: '*Every stottery cow wants a friend.*'

But, as always happens, a new supplier soon fills the gap in the market left by the old. What is bought and sold as 'heroin' once again contains heroin. In Toronto there was a terrible spate of drug-related deaths. Users, unaware that their product had been cut to zero, had lost their tolerance, and didn't know to adjust their dose. When they went on injecting their usual bag, back to full strength now, they fell like trees, stopped breathing, suffocated on their vomit.

———

Another post card from Pakistan:
    On the hill above Skardu there was a UN monitoring station. I climbed up to it, one afternoon, curious about the aerials and

satellite dishes, and keen to talk to someone, anyone, who wasn't a Muslim man from the Punjab.

The station was manned by a young Australian soldier only a year or two older than myself. He had been there for weeks, and seemed utterly unconcerned by his isolation.

He offered me tea and offered me 'something stronger'. In a diplomatic shed round the back, he had a tiny brewery, a bubbling kit of yeast and hops and barley secretly sustained by the generations of young Australians rotating through. I spent the afternoon drinking strong, cloudy beer. I hadn't had alcohol for three months, and somewhere at the back of my head I worried about my tolerance, but I didn't want to seem rude. He asked me, in passing, whether I would be prepared to spy for the UN: perhaps see my way to reporting numbers of casualties, levels of gunshot wounds, evidence of unusual intensification of the fighting among my military hosts? But I declined. That would be a kind of betrayal. The soldier said 'No worries, mate!' and we fell to talking about rugby, climbing and girls.

I stumbled home in the evening, cold, drunk, feeling watched and judged, though nothing was said by anyone. I fell into my bed and was sick that night, and ill the next day. My hosts shook their heads and said 'Jalluhb' (dysentery), and had the cook prepare me sweet bland food like custard, putting my illness down to too much chilli for my western stomach. That was a low: a miserably lonely point.

I tend to the socially liberal, on just about everything.

Without thinking about it too carefully, without really committing, I've suspected for ages that the criminal justice system's persecution of drug users has just had the effect of making everything worse, for everyone. Then, a couple of years ago, I went to a talk by the journalist Johann Hari about his book, *Chasing the Scream*, at the Edinburgh book festival. Hari is a charismatic speaker: fiercely bright, articulate, clear, passionate, convincing. I queued up after to talk with him, which is a thing I almost never do. I queued for over an hour, and when it was my turn at last, as happens, just splurged, 'Your book, it's changed my life!' which it had, and does, but I was number 200 in a long line of fans, and the man was glazed over and tired. He shook my hand and smiled, wished me well, and signed my copy of his book.

Hari argues that the war against drugs, at least in the US, is a race war, but by a different name. That it started as an employment strategy for agents of the US Agency for Firearms, Alcohol and Tobacco, whose jobs were threatened in the 1920s by the repeal of prohibition, and then, almost immediately doubled up as a tool for the oppression of black culture; at the time heroin was the favoured tipple for black musicians. He states as an iron law, that prohibition leads to the maximum concentration and potency of the prohibited substance. He cites coca leaf and cocaine; opium and heroin; beer and the blinding 'white lightning' that appeared in the US at the time of prohibition, and disappeared as soon as prohibition was repealed.

It's prohibition itself that leads to most drug-related harms. In those countries, such as Portugal, where heroin users are tolerated and are provided with safe facilities for injecting, heroin deaths almost disappear. In those countries where prohibition is repealed, there is a modest bump in substance misuse, and massive reduction in substance-related harm.

Hari tells the story of an undercover police officer in a US inner city who is monitoring the activities of a group of 'hoppers', adolescent boys who use push bikes to shuttle between street level drug dealers and a central depot, so that the street dealer is never carrying more than a small, disposable amount of narcotic at any one time. One of the children approaches the police officer, offers him money to go into a local shop, asks that he buy him alcohol. The police officer declines, noting that the child is carrying on him hundreds of dollars' worth of pills and powder, but still needs to ask a grownup to buy booze. When substances are prohibited, the regulation of their production and sale reverts from the state to gangsters and children.

The book introduced me to the famous 'Rat Park'. Rat Park was an experiment conducted in the late seventies by Canadian psychologist Bruce K. Alexander. Alexander sought to undermine the traditional view that it was the narcotic that caused addiction. He repeated the Skinner box experiment with populations of caged rats, addicted them to morphine, but then varied the scenario. He demolished the cages and built for them instead an alternative environment: a rat paradise, with plenty of space, plenty of wheels to run around, wood to gnaw on, balls, tunnels and platforms for the rats to play on, lots of opposite sex rats, and private spaces for rat families to grow and thrive. There was as much morphine available as in the Skinner boxes, but none of the rats showed any propensity for addictive behaviour. A few tried the morphine, a few returned to it, but there was no problematic drug use.

Addicted rats, moved from their cramped Skinner boxes into 'Rat Park', rapidly re-socialised, found mates, had pups, rapidly stopped preferring the morphine bottles to the food. A few twitched and shivered for a bit, but soon settled. There were no problems with withdrawal. It seems that it wasn't the morphine causing the problem after all; and their addiction certainly wasn't the fault of the rats. It was the cages all along. Odd though, how the long science of rats in cages, and rats in parks, has served over the years to construct the phenomena it purports to explain.

Nonetheless: the law isn't helping.

Though Derek would disagree.

———

Derek's involvement with the law goes back to babyhood. He knows what he's talking about. He was born in London, but his mother, who was in and out of prison, was unable to look after him, and so he was adopted by a Scottish couple. By some mystery of genes or culture, he has kept his accent. He sounds like Sid James. He sounds like a Cockney character in a 1950s comedy. Sometimes I think he puts it on for effect.

Derek is resilient. Derek's a survivor. *He* had no enabling mother to keep him fed and housed – and thus alive, for long enough for his body to rot like Mikey's.

The adoption failed. I read his notes. He had unmanageable behavioural problems, so he went into care, and then a succession of foster homes – fostered long enough to break the hearts of the new parents, but never contained for long enough to thrive – then back into care for the final stretch, and then the world.

Derek has been buying and selling drugs for as long as he can remember. He has had few options having missed school, not a hope of a job, and no work ethic anyway – how would he have a work ethic? – then the blight of an early prison sentence. That's him set. He started with glue, then small amounts of grass, MDMA, heroin, of course, cocaine when possible, lots of speed.

Derek is slippery and dodgy, but he has a bit of banter to him. He once took a call on his mobile when he was in my surgery room. He was in with a penile discharge. I thought he had the clap (gonorrhea), and was poised to take a swab, when his phone went. This was early in the first phase of our relationship, way back, years ago. He flashed me a little smile, pointed with his finger at the screen, mouthed the words 'Do you mind, Doc?' Which I do! God, I really do! I shook my head and hissed, but he took the call anyway. People always seem to. I'm about to show him the door, tackle out or not, when I find myself distracted and deflated by the end of his call.

'… tiny little place, you'll not miss it … tenner bags … okay … okay … fine, plenty! … You'll have it all mind? … okay, but don't let me down pal! … yep, okay!. … cheerio then, luvya!'

'Luvya?' I say, curious, realising I have misunderstood how this kind of relationship works. It's clearly not at all like it is on the telly.

'Sure,' he says, roguishly, 'Old friend. Old, old friend.'

Derek is whip thin and younger than his years: dyed black hair, skinny faded jeans, black ankle boots, tightly muscled, clean and well tattooed. I suspect he carries a blade, but he leaves it at the door when he comes to see me. He's all smile and wit and charm when he comes to see me.

'I've always had the greatest respect for doctors. You guys work your arses off to get to where you get to!'

My relationship with Derek has occupied two distinct phases. The first, over a three-or-four year period, interspersed by brief periods in prison, when I would see him every month for a prescription for methadone: a low, unchanging dose, occasionally he would have heroin in his urine, occasionally cocaine, but he seemed unconcerned by it. He didn't see his drug use as a problem, as such, just a way of life, so in that sense, none of my concern really. The methadone kept him well, kept him on a level and free from temptation. It meant, I suspect, that he didn't need to dip into his own supply. Is this a legitimate purpose for medicine? I don't know really. I suspect it is. But I suspect most people would disagree. Derek, in the second phase of our relationship, certainly disagreed. Derek, back then, had resilience and bounce and charm, and I didn't judge him. I didn't *need* to judge him: he always treated me with respect. Then young Derek disappeared. Young Derek died.

Four years passed, the same Derek pitches up, but old now. Dyed black hair all gone, his scalp is shaved, and no longer fit, or quick, or lean, and the face is lined and sun-damaged. I can see now how he'll age. He has a deep suntan.

'Haven't seen you for a long, long time!'

'I've been away!'

'Holiday?' I ask stupidly.

'You could say so … long holiday, Belize, care of Her Majesty…'

'Ah…'

A word to potential drug smugglers:

According to Derek, Caribbean airport customs get junior staff from British embassies to stand with them, once or twice a week, to help to pick out the large numbers of low-level drug mules trying to take advantage of the easy-going cocaine trade active in that part of the world. According to Derek, who is, admittedly, in most areas, highly unreliable, the local customs officials complain that *these people all look the same to them:* they don't find it so easy to pick out the fiends from the family holidaymakers. The embassy staff can do it in an instant. For them, it's a bit of a laugh, according to Derek. The one who picked him out was perfectly polite, even slightly apologetic. 'English guy. You'll know the type. Suit. Oxbridge chap, bit of a wanker, nice enough though.'

'You've been in prison? For four years?'

As I say, Derek is resilient.

'Yep – shared cell. Concrete floor, nothing to sleep on but a mat. That's why I've come to see you: I think I may have done something to my back…' And it's true – he is standing a little oddly.

'Shared cell…?'

He grimaces. Bats away a bad memory. 'Sure … but nothing I'm not used to. It was just like being back in care again!'

Right. Resilient.

'Methadone?'

He raises his hand and shakes his head. 'Defi-nate-ly not! No-thank-you, Doctor! Four years free! Don't want any more of your methadone or any other crap. No way, hos-ay. Not a chance. Prison's set me free of that…'

I wait for the scam. There is no scam.

'So how did you stop?'

Derek had been on a prescription for methadone for 15 years, and whenever he was released from Scottish prisons, he'd need a little more. He had never shown the slightest interest in stopping before.

'Well, I had to. I was in a cell...'

'And?'

He laughs at my ignorance.

'It's not like here. It's a good job being a prison guard in Belize. You get paid well. There aren't any drugs in Belize prisons, not even weed. It's a question of professional pride for them: the guards just won't stand for it.'

Right.

Derek is more transformed than anyone that I have ever met. He has put on weight in the years since his return, lost his hair and most of his looks. He has married a girl much younger than himself, Loti, from the Czech Republic, and they have a baby, whom they fret over: whenever the child is sick, or has a cold or a rash, they bring her in. It's charming, in its way, given the story.

I see most of my drug addict patients on a Tuesday afternoon. It suits me better to have them all together – more manageable. Derek and Loti have been waiting for an hour or so to see me, while I work my way through my clinic, running late as usual. When I call them through, Derek puffs a bit when he stands. He has a bit of a fat person's waddle, and I think *he's letting himself go.* He jabs a finger at his watch, charmlessly, as they come through, and as they sit down he says, 'I see you're still in the drug-dealing business, Doc!' which *really* riles me. Loti undresses the child, cooing as she does, and it strikes me that she knows nothing at all about her husband's past.

'Lock the fuckers up, I say, and throw away the key. It's the only thing that works…'

'*Derek!* Ze child!' says Loti, covering the infant's ears, and Derek smirks. Contentment has been bad for Derek.

I find myself missing the man I used to know.

———

Listen to Gale.

She has been addicted to heroin for almost as long as she can remember. And the time *before* that, is a time so painful, she won't think about it. She resents being asked to try.

The thought of being free of drugs, is painful too. Gale can hardly imagine a world without that protective veil.

From my perspective, none of this is Gale's fault: she is as the world has determined. It would be inhuman to *blame* her. She has made choices, true, but none of these has really been *hers* to make. It is as if Gale has no agency: no control over her own world.

On the other hand … if, to be considered an adult in the world, a person has to make decisions for themselves, own these decisions, and seek to be as free as possible to make these things called choices, then Gale, in that important sense, is scarcely an adult at all. And if, to seek freedom and agency in the world is an important attribute of personhood, then, in that sense, Gale scarcely counts as a person. To be fair to Gale, she wouldn't see things in that way, not at all. Gale would hate the implication: she'd punch it right back, and quite right too. And I don't see *myself* in that light either. From where I stand, *I* make choices all the time, and they're mine and no one else's. Illusion or not, whether it makes any sense to an outsider, it's how the world feels to me, and how I want it to be: to be a thing that makes choices, that's part of what makes living precious. It's part of what makes me a person. And, thinking about it, that's how I treat friends and family as well – *as if* they were persons, as if they were things that made decisions and choices too, as if they valued these things, just as much as I do. That seems like a question of respect. The most basic kind of respect.

Another paradox of heroin: nothing is ever your fault, yet, *everything* is your fault.

It's not just a paradox of heroin.

All of this matters. Not least because I see Gale every fourth Tuesday afternoon, and if I'm to follow through on this commitment, I need a plan. I need a cohesive, practical theory, that works.

The theory is this: In every interaction that I have with Gale, my duty is to try to act in such a way as to increase her agency. To increase her capacity to make the kinds of choices that the best version of herself would make.

This entails:

+ Turning up. Listening to her. Not fading out. Not engaging in epic daydreams;
+ Not colluding with her drug use. Not *expecting* it;
+ Being incredibly paternalistic (She's *42*! But doing this anyway);
+ Encouraging conversation about the 'best version of Gale'. Acknowledging how that conversation hurts, but powering on through;

+ Being nice to her when she's nice to me, and chilly when she's not;
+ Making a relationship with her and using that relationship as a tool for change;
+ Listening to her talk about her new dog. Seem interested. It emerges that the best version of Gale is the one that looks after animals. She walks her new dog every day, clearly loves him, cares for him – this is encouraging;
+ Reduce her methadone, bit by bit, since she's no longer using heroin. Since she stopped using heroin, she's looking better: clean, better dressed, teeth fixed. (Getting your teeth fixed is an investment in a future. Good sign, I think.)

She gets down to 3ml daily of methadone, then gets stuck. But that's *nothing! You* wouldn't notice 3ml of methadone!

Her tolerance for opiates drops to nothing too. I forget to discuss this detail with her.

————

Back in the late eighties I worked in A&E in a small town in Lancashire. The medicine was fun, though frightening. During my first couple of shifts on nights, I was supervised by Ronald, an ex-army charge nurse with blue tinted glasses and a wispy moustache, who called me 'Sir'. There were no other doctors as such during that first week. Ronald sat smoking in the nurse's tea room with the other nurses while I saw the patients, helped by an Indian nursing auxiliary called Izzie. When we saw a patient that Izzie and I couldn't handle – a fractured femur, say, that needed splinting – I'd call Ronald through, and ask him in my shaky young voice, 'How exactly do you … ah … splint a fractured femur?' and Ronald would respond, bracingly, 'You're in charge, Sir,' with a kind of resentful smirk, and wait for my instructions. He made me feel like the posh young lieutenant on his first day in the trenches, losing his head.

What a bunch these nurses were! What a coven. Ronald (Sir!) with his snake-thin hips and crappy moustache, and Heather with her knitting and Players No6 that she kept in a jewelled cigarette case with little snappy clips. She talked about 'Pakis' (she 'hated Pakis') and when there was a death from that community, and the public corridors would fill with the wailing of bereaved, she'd clip her mouth tight shut and shake her head in disgust and say, 'They're not like us … Pakis…' That was what the world was like in 1989. Heather, I think, will be dead by now.

On night four I was napping in the relatives' room when there was tapping on the door, and someone poked their head round and said, 'Do you want a cuppa, Pete?'

I don't much like being called 'Pete', but I liked John, especially as he showed me the way to the night canteen and introduced me to Wendy, the jolly night-shift cook, who cooked us a mid-night breakfast while we sat and drank tea and chatted. Loneliness, and the long night-time hours spent in a rainy town near Wigan, had made me porous, and, besides, John was younger, brighter, had been around the world a bit, and thought that Ronald was a twat. I choked with laughter and relief; hot brown tea came shooting down my nose, as can happen.

John had trained as a nurse, but wanted to be a musician. He'd lived for years in a squat in Berlin, written some songs, been on the radio a few times, learned German. I had a friend, Gordon, best friend at school, who had followed the same trajectory. John thought perhaps that he had known him. We talked about hanging out in squats in Berlin, drinking beer, watching the swans drifting on the lakes and the young folks dressed in black, rolling by on bikes.

'So why did you…'

'Come back?'

'Yeah.'

'Married now. Two kids. Respectability called!'

Later, there was a crash call: a young woman came in, blue, scarcely breathing, eyes wide with panic and the immediacy of death, and John, who had seen it all before, nodded and said, 'Tension pneumothorax. Ever done a chest drain, Pete?' I shook my head, and John said, 'First time then!'

And John sat by her head as the girl stretched herself out, arms reaching to his, as he comforted her, whilst saying to me, 'Left side!' and 'Between the third and fourth intercostal space, over the rib, not under … that's right…' And as I threatened to push too hard bayonet-style on the metal introducer, said, 'Not too hard … There you go, love, we're in…' (to the girl), and breathed, 'Well done, Pete, high five…' as we reviewed the chest x-ray after, saw the plastic chest drain sitting in the right spot, the lung re-inflating, and the girl, all pink now though shaken up, being wheeled to the ward.

A few months later, there was another crash call. A man, 32 years old, found by his wife collapsed at home. Not breathing say the ambulance crew enroute. They think it's an overdose, likely heroin. I know what I'm doing, by this stage. I take the head end, which is the technical bit, and my colleague the chest compressions. I ask her to stop a moment, while I open the man's mouth, stabilise the chin, thrust the jaw forward, introduce a laryngoscope, view the larynx and the vocal cords, suck out vomit from the trachea, introduce a laryngeal tube, connect it to oxygen, 100 per cent, noting as I pass, the smell of alcohol and vomit, the dilated pupils, the pallor of his lips, the sheen of sweat, new coldness gathering on the man's skin.

'I think he's dead,' says my colleague after a bit. 'I think we should stop.'

'Me too,' I say, noting the puncture mark in the crook of the left elbow, which neither my colleague nor myself had made. Bits of history have filtered through to us from the relatives' room. He had been off drugs for years, his wife had told the nursing staff. Then, an unwelcome visitor, an old friend from his past, turned up. They'd had a couple of beers, maybe a joint. They were sat listening to their music. She had no idea.

There was wailing in the corridor when we stopped. The wife, the kids. Heather with her mouth clipped tight shut.

'Have you seen the name on the card, Sir?' says Ronald, later, with a smirk, because I clearly haven't clocked what's happened yet.

I hadn't recognised him. It was John, the nurse-musician from Berlin. His face was upside down so I didn't really get to see him. And besides, the dead look different.

———

'Doctor?' says Gale.

I've drifted off again. A sad memory, dropping in, visiting me of its own accord, like an old friend from the past. I shake myself back into the here and now. It doesn't bother Gale at all, these absences of mine. I wouldn't say that we were like old friends exactly, but there is a kind of comfort to our relationship now, which is rare and precious. 3ml of methadone! For three years! We laugh about it, but she just can't get any lower, she gets withdrawals. However 'in her head' they are, as I point out to her, they're real enough for Gale.

She has a little dog-walking business. She dresses fine, in an outdoorsy kind of way, and hasn't used heroin for 18 months, which is a record.

'There's something I've been meaning to discuss with you…'

She raises her eyebrows. *I'm listening…*

'It's about your tolerance – the risk of overdose…'

'I'm never going to use again, Doctor, don't you worry!'

'Sure,' I say, 'but if you do…'

When Darkness Falls

Joy remembered that when she was very little a young man would sometimes come to the tenement flat where she lived with her mother and her father and younger brother, and he would take her out to the drying green at the back of the block, to play. She looked forward to his visits. He made a fuss of her: he treated her in a special way – hoisting her onto his shoulders and striding out with her like that, hoisted aloft as if she were the rider and he her great brute shire horse, and he would neigh and whinny and kick his legs, and she would laugh and scream out loud, begging him to stop/begging him to carry on. She remembered how the coarse material of his uniform would scratch at her bare legs and make them itch. She remembered his cropped hair and the sweet smell of hair oil. The uniform dates it, she thinks, and the little kit bag that he would leave by the front door by the hat stand when he came a-clattering in and shouted 'I'm here!'. She would have been three or four years old. It would have been the early 1940s, it would have had to be, but she didn't know for sure. She didn't know where he was stationed, whether he fought, whether he had a good or a bad war, or anything much really about what had happened to him in his young life.

She remembered that her father called him Jim, and Jim called her father 'Dad', and she remembered how her mother, Betty, an austere, humourless woman, would cool yet more when Jim came to stay. Even as a tiny child she was aware that Jim brought with him his own atmosphere. There was distance between these two: Betty, not so many years older than Jim, disappeared into herself when he visited. She could tell how this pained her much older father and how he longed to make a home to welcome this stranger who was, presumably, his son.

She could never talk for long about Jim without becoming distressed. Something would coil up inside her as she told the story. It would start well enough. She would brighten, and talk lyrically about that strong sense memory: the cold air outside, the dank passage leading out to the drying green, her pink bare legs scratching on the woollen serge of his army uniform, the sheen of his hair, and that sense, rare and intoxicating to a small child, of being sought out and wanted. But that joy in physical recollection would cloud quickly.

'I knew how much my mother hated Jim's visits. However hard she tried, she still hated them, and she couldn't hide it. And then he stopped coming, and I never knew why. They wouldn't talk about it. There were always so many secrets. Then, after dad died, there was no possibility of asking.'

'So what happened to Jim?'

'I heard nothing more about him. As an older child, then when I was growing up, he just never came back. I had always wondered who he was, where he fitted in, why he called dad "Dad". The penny only really dropped when I was grown up, when I had you, when I first got ill, and started thinking about these things again. Isn't that odd? How children are? And that my mother was jealous of him, or ashamed, or whatever it was. Whatever in the world could there be to be so ashamed of?'

'What happened to Jim?'

She cries. Her son waits for her to stop. Her son, who ordinarily has no problem expressing love to those he loves, seems to struggle to take her hand, but he does. Her hand sits there, like a bundle of dry twigs in his.

'A few years before mum died I got a letter from a hospital in England. It was a mental hospital, actually. He had been there for a long time. It seems that Jim hadn't had a happy life. I think he may have become alcoholic, reading between the lines. He had heard somehow that I was a lawyer, and wanted to make me next of kin. I don't think that he had anyone else. I don't know how he got my address.'

She cries some more. She takes a sip of tea from the beaker on the push-in table in front of her, coughs, swallows. Her hand is shaking a little. There are scraps of food everywhere. Cold nursing-home soup, drying bread and butter, a slice of cake, untouched. She has stopped eating; she has lost a great deal of weight. To eat is torture; to try to make her eat is even worse. The tea steadies her.

'What did you do?'

'Mum was still alive, and I had you two to worry about. It just wasn't something that I could deal with then. Your father didn't want me to get involved, and my mother would have been just terribly upset, so I didn't do anything. I didn't reply. I threw the letter away. I regret it terribly now. It was the only thing left in the world of your uncle Jim.'

Her son nods, startled a little by his mother's turn of phrase, not previously having considered the possibility that this ghost from the past, this lost soldier, of whom it seems no trace in the world remains, had any real connection with him.

'I didn't hear anything more for a couple of years, and then I got a short note from the hospital, just to say that he had died. I don't know what he died from. I have this idea that it may have been suicide, but I don't know. And by that time mum had died anyway. He had no personal possessions. It was a terrible wrong. I threw his letter away.'

Joy had lived a blessed kind of life, by any standard, although she came from some poverty. *Her* mother, Betty, had had no education and had worked in a jute mill as a child, just like previous generations of mothers. Her father came from some privilege – from grand people living in grand houses – but something had gone wrong in his life. He was practically blind, either as a consequence of a schoolyard accident, a blow to the head from a stone in a snowball, or because he was gassed in the trenches; it was never clear. He was a passionate communist, temperance man, stalwart trade unionist. He worked as a carpenter down at the docks, but couldn't retain work consistently; the blindness and the activist politics being, then and now, impediments to employability. By the time he married Betty, late in life, already in his sixties, he had slid into unemployment and poverty, both sustained and thwarted by his pride. What did the young Betty see in the blind old man? Why did she choose *him*, or let herself be chosen? He was a good man, though, in his heart. Joy remembered her father always as striving to be a certain kind of a man: a worker, a provider, a sober strong man. She remembered him as fumbling and incontinent and blind and hopeless, and she remembered being embarrassed and ashamed by his brokenness, by his age, and she remembered her mother's shame too. But when she was a small child he used to take her to political meetings. She remembered being caught in an air-raid on the way back home from a meeting of the local party. She remembered the darkness, searchlights, a pure kind of exhilaration; being in the company of her father, being shepherded into a public shelter that smelled of sweat and tea, sitting there in a fug of warmth and damp tweed, waiting for those bombs to come raining down.

She described a curious sense that she had always had of having been born into the wrong life. As a small child, she spoke differently from others around her. Strangers in the street would draw attention to the fact of how well the little girl spoke, how pure and English were her vowels, at a time when manner of speech was life determining, but she was teased for it at school. Although she could be condescending, she wasn't a snob – but she was a stranger in her community. She was clever. She was very musical. Though untaught, she learned to play the piano, and then the organ, and when she was older, intolerant of her native poverty, she paid her way through school and then university by playing the organ in church and taking the church choir. Her sons thought that there was heroism in this. Despite everything that came later, she was always admired and loved, although she could never understand that.

When she was 11 her life changed: she won a scholarship to the local high school, the fee-paying school where she was taught Greek, was given voice coaching, where she learned to sing Schubert Lieder and light opera, where she was nurtured. She won a scholarship to the Royal Academy of Music to sing, but she didn't take it, choosing instead to study law in her home city, where she met the man who became her husband.

She felt an outsider at home; she felt an imposter at school, at university, in the law. When she was 12, she had had to make her own school uniform, running up skirts and blouses on the treadle sewing machine in her mother's front room. It was her secret to make copies, exact copies, of the clothes her new friends wore freshly purchased from the department store in the centre of town where her parents couldn't shop, to make exact copies so that no one would know they weren't bought.

The man she married was a doctor's son. His family welcomed her into the big house with the surgery on the ground floor in the part of town on the green by the river where she had scarcely previously visited. They welcomed her. They admired her singing and her playing, and were pleased that their clever, shy son had found this sweet girl who so evidently made him happy. They fitted one another. He played the piano for her, she sang to her new family. They welcomed her into the house. When he left to complete his national service, she stayed in the doctor's house by the river, and learned to cook and bake, taught by her mother-in-law to be, who sensed something vulnerable in the child who was going to be her daughter-in-law, and made it her business to care for her as if she were her own child. She welcomed that warmth and recognised their kindness, but couldn't rid herself of the fear that she would be found out. The safer she was, it seemed, the greater the jeopardy. She was always on her guard, vigilant, but against what she could never say. She couldn't rid herself of the sense – the truth underlying – that this life wasn't her life to keep, that it was provisional, undeserved, that it would all end.

He returned from the army, changed, but for the better. He had a disfiguring port-wine stain which had precluded serving as an officer, and so, the shy doctor's boy had been thrown to the ranks where he had survived the name calling from which he had previously always been protected. He learned, as he put it awkwardly, to get on with common people. He was confident, less shy, had ended up serving abroad, working as secretary to a general in Fontainebleau. They married. After a couple of miscarriages, she had two sons, and they lived in a little house in the small town where he had work as an administrator in a university.

Her son has heard these stories many, many times before. He has grown tired of the resentment that has grown over the years in his mother, directed against all these people who have tried so hard, for so long, to love her. All those who have understood her, and have tried to make the bad thing, whatever it was, go away! Although he knows this is unfair, he feels this fierce resentment of hers to be directed at him. Bitterness is hard to be around. She starts on again, intoning the same threnody. Her son is ungenerous.

'Your father never understood what it was to be poor. He had everything given to him; I had to work for it. I had to work. I played the organ every Sunday, then choir in the evening, then study, and he *never* understood.'

She circles round and around the same stories. There is one that she always returns to:

'It was as if, one day, suddenly, from nowhere, darkness fell.'

ii

On some days it can seem that every other patient that I see is complaining of unhappiness. I try not to use the word 'depression', or at least I try not to be the first. Unhappiness is what we feel – from the most minor, delicate grey-shaded garment that clings to our skin when we wake in the morning, the flimsy thing we shrug off like our night-clothes, all the way through to a muddy shroud that wraps and suffocates, the cold wet from its folds seeping through us so that we smell of its fabric. Worthlessness. Shame. Unhappiness has always been with us, in all of its different colours and degrees.

'Depression' is a new word for an old thing. It's a label, and one which carries with it its own baggage of meanings and associations. A portmanteau word, it's a closed bag whose contents can remain hidden and unexamined. It is a word that is at times immensely useful, descriptive, powerful in its effect. It's also a word to be cautious of, like any powerful agent in the world.

'Unhappiness' is, perhaps, less complicated. Less loaded. More purely descriptive. More specific.

I first met Maddison a few years ago. She would have been about 11. She came to see me with her mother. A fairly adult 11. She was tall for her age, had thick brown hair pulled back in an Alice band, skin unblemished and pre-pubertal, tight leggings, little patent leather sandals, a tight but not immodest top. A very poised child, she seemed to me, a child becoming aware of how she appears in the world, to others. Hard time of life. She looked at her feet and let her mother do the talking.

'We've become very moody in the last few months, haven't we, Maddy? We've had a bit of bullying, and quite a few tantrums at home, quite a few bedroom doors being slammed. Madam's becoming quite hard to live with.'

'I see.'

Maddison's eyes tear into the carpet at her feet.

'*And* we've got some pretty important exams coming up, don't we, Maddison?'

Her mother looks at me, meaningfully. I don't really understand what it is she's getting at, but then I often don't.

'... then this morning we didn't want to go to school, and then Maddison disclosed something. Tell the doctor what you disclosed. Look at the doctor, Maddison.'

Maddison's knuckles are white, clutching at her pink smartphone. Her eyes are gripped shut, her face like a clenched fist, she shakes her head and squeezes out two tears which shake onto the carpet like scattered raindrops.

'Maddison disclosed that she has been having thoughts about self harming,' her mother says solemnly, tears now in *her* eyes.

You can see the child in the mother. She has the same rich, chestnut hair, a well-cut business suit, a hint of tobacco behind the fragrant soap and face cream. Keys to the Audi and a smartphone, still on, on the table between us. She is in her late thirties and fit; she diets ruthlessly to keep fit. They have taken my first Monday morning slot, 7.30 a.m., and Maddison's mum has already been to the gym. She looks tense, anxious, so, so tired.

I happen to know, although Maddison presumably doesn't, that her mother is being treated with antidepressants, prescribed by a colleague; that last year she had been signed off work after several months of work-related stress caused by bullying by her line manager. She works as a manager in an insurance office, one that has its headquarters at the other side of town. She is a link in a very long, weight-bearing chain. She fears that if she takes more time off sick, she will be replaced. Maddison attends a little private primary school. They live in an old Victorian house on the shores of the loch. When I cycle to work in the morning, I can see the grey stones rising out of the mist by the water.

They have everything! The woman's life still sounds like a grind.

I happen to know, though Maddison's mother presumably doesn't, that her husband has a problem with gambling. He is an overbearing man with a crushingly loud voice, who works in the same company, in finance, and earns in bonuses what I do in a year. He is away a lot. He spends too much time on the internet, and has a private prescription for Viagra. But all that, I think, is another matter.

'Self harming, Maddie?'

I look at Maddie. I avoid looking at her mother. I want the child to speak for herself, though how to achieve that I haven't really got a clue.

Maddie peeps up. A little brown eye squints up from under her masses of brown hair. She catches my eye, looks again at her feet.

'Self harming, Maddie?'

Two quick nods. The little brown eye glances up, holds mine a second or two longer.

'She's been jabbing this into her leg.' Her mother produces from her bag an antique brass letter opener.

'Did you break the skin, Maddie?'

Two quick shakes of the head.

'She left a bruise though ... Show the doctor your leg, Maddie.'

The child jumps suddenly to her feet, strips down her legging, and shows me a bruise on her leg. It's nothing.

'Why did you do that, Maddie?'

'I don't know.'

At least she's talking to me now.

'Are you a bit unhappy, Maddie?'

She bites her lower lip, nods a couple of times. The willowy young woman with the cascade of chestnut hair has been put aside for a moment. She's reverted to childhood.

'Why's that?'

'I don't know.'

A boy in her class is being mean to her. Boys once shouted and spat in the playground, pushed in, in lunch queues, swore and farted and wiped snot on the girls' stuff when the teacher wasn't looking. Boys were vile. *This* boy, though, has been sending Maddie bad texts and rude photographs. She doesn't like it. Teachers once dealt with bullying by physically separating the protagonists. But the bad boy's texts cross all of space effortlessly, and always: at home, school, on holiday, there's no escaping the little pink phone.

There have been changes in Maddie's friendship group in school; some girls that were her friends are no longer. They are older girls for their age, and one of them smokes. The word 'slag' has been used. Maddie says she doesn't want to be friends with them anymore, although I suspect she probably does. It all seems connected with the texts, but the child won't be separated from her phone, day or night, whatever her mother says. But Maddie has one good mate still – a boy, an old playmate, as it happens – and whenever Maddie feels stressed in class, she simply has to put up her hand, and her friend, in whom she confides, will take her to the 'safe place' until she feels ready to go back.

I bring Maddie back to see me. On the second visit the phone is gone and to my surprise she chats to me and occasionally smiles. Her mother, at first, had wanted something to be done, and quick, about Maddie's moods. She had mentioned this, but in a roundabout kind of way, too polite to demand, but worried, nonetheless, by my slowness to respond to something which to her was so obvious.

'Isn't there a tablet you can use? Isn't there something that we can give her? To calm her down? Cheer her up?'

Unstated *Like the one I'm on…*

Her mother thinks that there is a tablet, or a cure, for her daughter's unhappiness. Right or wrong, her mother has good reason to think this way.

There is a default way in which these kinds of conversations can go, at least with adults. After a brief investigation of symptoms, sleep hygiene, alcohol, suicidality and self-harm risk, and the filling out of a facile symptom questionnaire which takes about two minutes and tells me nothing I didn't know already, without care and attention, the consultation with the unhappy person will drift towards a prescription for an anti-depressant – an SSRI like Prozac usually, or something else. These conversations run like trains on fixed rails, hammered together by drugs manufacturers and their doctors. It takes considerable time and effort for the conversation to go otherwise, and for it to do so I have to lift against gravity: my limited time, my limited resources, ingrained patient expectations and deeper social conventions. It means that I also have to take risks. It's always safer in medicine to do what's expected of you. If people want a tablet, it feels safer, easier and quicker just to give it. And it's almost always wrong. But people can have deep expectations of the power of what they think of as science. Maddie's mother has somehow come to understand her emotions in these terms. She understands her daughter's so, too.

I think *You're teaching your daughter how to be unhappy, in the same way that you are unhappy*. But there aren't any words to express such a thought, at least none that I can find, that aren't cruel or just stupid.

And today Maddie seems a little better to me. She seems less guarded. She still says she hates school, but seems less committed to the view. She acknowledges with a grudging smile that her teacher is kind of nice. She spends less time in the 'safe space' and more time in class and is doing well. In the evening she has started dancing classes with her friend. Her teacher and her mother want me to refer Maddie to Children's and Adolescent Mental Health Services. I broach the subject with Maddie.

'Are you still hurting yourself, Maddie?'

She is sucking on a lock of hair. She shakes her head hurriedly. Her mother stares at her daughter through narrow, angry eyes.

'Sometimes I think about it though…'

'Okay,' I say, 'But it's no longer quite so … tempting?'

Shakes her head.

'Your mum and Ms Rainer were thinking it might help if we were to ask a specialist to talk with you, about how you're feeling. I think that that might help too…'

She looks doubtful. She senses something insincere.

'Sometimes it can help to talk with an expert about how you're feeling. Sometimes an expert can help you make sense of what it is you're feeling, especially if you're feeling bad. If you're thinking about self-harming, for example…'

But can that possibly make sense? To an 11-year-old? Would it have made any sense to me, as an 11-year-old?

'How long would that take, Doctor?' asks her mother.

'About…'

Three months? Six months? Even longer? And what would I write anyway? That this bright kid, this sensitive kid, was thinking of jabbing a letter opener into her leg, but she changed her mind?

'About … well, there *would* be a bit of a wait…'

'Right…'

Maddie's mother thinks that there is a comprehensive system, a structure which can be accessed, that will have the skill and training and knowledge to know how to fix Maddie. It's true, there *is* a system, although I'm pretty sure that it wouldn't claim to 'fix' anyone, but also it is utterly and completely overwhelmed by people like Maddie. The greater the provision of service grows, the greater the problem grows, and who knows here what is cause and what is effect? The problem of child and adolescent mental health is a hydra-headed monster. The service doesn't keep up. It can seem as if all this talk there is in the world about mental health serves to fuel the thing that is talked about.

'What do *you* think, Maddie?'

I think that she is standing on the verge of a defining decision, and one that I fear she will return to in life. That there has opened up at her feet a whole diverse world of intriguing, bleak new possibilities: of swirling dark, purple moods, the beguiling razor, the attention of whisper-voiced adults like me who ask solicitously after her thoughts, digging for feelings, rooting out her pain.

Maddie looks long and hard at her feet and shudders; looks up, squints at me as if there is light shining in her face. I have this sense that Maddie, wiser than her years, has looked deep into this dark forest of possibilities.

She shakes her head. '*Nah.*' Not for now, at least.

The last time I saw Maddie, she had seemed brighter. She was spending her free time dancing with her friend. She no longer cared for those other, bad friends who had dropped her, and the bad boy and his texts are forgotten. She smiled and said 'thank-you' unprompted when she left, although I hadn't done anything much at all. Things seemed a little better for Maddie; sometimes things just blow over. Things seemed better, at least for now.

iii
It was as if one day, suddenly, from nowhere, darkness fell.

She would describe the tyranny of being a house-mother in the early sixties. She had given up her work as a lawyer when she had her two babies. She managed fine with the first, but something changed with the second.

She had internalised this punishing model of how it was to be done: how it involved an extraordinary, and unachievable, and undesirable, level of perfection. Of washing, and ironing, of perfectly functioning, perfectly turned out babies, and a clean welcoming house, a punishing schedule of home baking and cooking, and the maintenance of a sunny outlook on life – a certain quality of coquettish smile, cheeriness and sophisticated up-beat humour, which was unsustainable. It was unclear where this pressure came from. Her mother-in-law was never unkind nor overtly demanding. Nor was her husband. Her children cried, but no more than other children. Her own mother had had no such expectations of herself, or of her daughter. It must have been in the air. In the *zeitgeist*. The break point came with a batch of scones that burned, and a second that also burned as her baby cried, and a third. At this point, a neighbour came by, concerned by the smell of smoke and a baby crying uncontrollably. They found her sitting immobilised on the kitchen floor as smoke poured from the oven, the baby crying in the cot, the older one sitting quietly, white faced and frightened, playing with his plastic soldiers in the corner of his bedroom. She mumbled to the neighbour through pale, pinched lips, '*Please call my husband.*'

'… from nowhere, darkness fell. I was in a fog. I couldn't see, I couldn't move, I couldn't do anything. I couldn't stop crying. I couldn't stop you from crying, or your brother from tugging at my sleeve and saying, "What's wrong, Mummy!"'

No one in these days knew what to do. They didn't know about depression then. She describes being taken in the little family car to the local mental hospital, but not knowing and not caring where she was being taken. She describes it as being a descent into hell – not that physical place where they took her, an institution where everyone seemed kind enough – but the place inside her own head, the place where she had taken herself. She blamed it on herself, of course.

'You don't understand the shame of it. Back then, it was just something that no one ever talked about.'

Her son, sitting on her nursing-home bed, listens to her talk. He wishes, wishes, wishes, that she would stop. These visits can be a torture. It's all so unpredictable. On a good day, he will take her out, they will eat pizza, she will flirt with the waiter, who is called Wojcek, and ask him about his home in Poland and he will be charmed. Then they will go home, to the family house, and watch a movie. 'Groundhog Day.' 'When Harry Met Sally.' He might play the violin for her and, if she is really well, she will pick out a ground bass and they will play Corelli, whose music she always loved. The cultured, intelligent woman, who could love life – that person whom others saw and knew – still lives in there, though she cowers and hides herself away most of the time, in terror and shame of her demon. But when she falls to talking about the bad things, those visits become interminable.

For years she never mentioned it. It was dimly understood by her sons that for a long period when they had been very small, she had been very unwell in hospital and that they had had to stay with their uncle and aunt, because their father, working, had been unable to cope alone with them. The older boy remembers it, the younger one not at all. For years she hadn't mentioned it – the sudden freeze, the catatonia, the descent into misery and inaction, the cold fog that fell in the middle of the day. She hadn't talked about it, but the fear of it, its unpredictability, its destructiveness, had governed her, more or less, throughout her life. It affected her relationship with her husband, who learned to fear her demon mood, and trod so quietly around her as a consequence, that the silence alone almost drove her mad. Her children learned never to do anything that might make her cry, because the crying might never end. Although it visited only intermittently, perhaps three or four times in her entire life, the snake-like shadow the demon cast was there always.

'You don't understand the shame of it. I wasn't allowed to see you for three months, and when I did, when they let your father bring you, you didn't recognise me. You pushed me away and started to cry. It was like you, even you, had rejected me. Even you were ashamed of me.'

Her son makes himself into a stone so that he doesn't flinch.

iv
Shame doesn't count as far as illness goes. Especially if it's deserved.

Another person came to see me with his unhappiness. Maddie's dad, as it happens: the tie and suit man in his late forties, the man with the money and the loud voice. He's carrying a load with him today, a big heavy burden. He slumps in his chair opposite, deposits it between us with a thud. A once muscled man now running fat, his white shirt strains. He sweats. He attempts a smile.

'Need a bit of help, Doctor.' The bass volume of his voice startles.

'Right.'

His medical notes are bare of clues. History of childhood illnesses, rugby injuries, a divorce, a subtle whiff of alcohol, but nothing much: nothing compared to some.

'Go on...?'

'It's the mood. It's shit.'

'Ah.' I nod and grunt.

Nod, grunt, wait, let him take you to the money.

'Been going on for weeks.'

'Weeks...?'

'Can't seem to shake it off and it's getting worse. Everyone's worried about me. Says I should get help.'

'Who's *everyone?*'

'My ... missus ... made me come.'

Mmm. Go on...?

And after a pause, to explain: 'She's gone to stay with her mum for a bit. Taken Maddie too. Too hard to be around ... me...'

'Ah...'

'So that's it, 49, on my own again!' Fake laugh. 'Fucked.' The head falls into the hands. The head jerks up again: '... says she wants the house though! Says I'll get fuck all!' He shakes his angry face.

Despair. Rage. Self pity. I don't warm to the combination.

'Oh dear.'

Pause. Wait. Wait. Wait. Then 'So things are a bit...'

'... shit. Yeah. I think I just need something to sleep, Doc. I'm tired all the time but I can't sleep. I've got *a lot* on at work. I think I need something to help me to sleep...'

'Sure. Okay ... maybe tell me ... what happened?'

'Work problems. Then the wife ups sticks. So Johnny here loses out. She wants the car as well! And now I can't sleep.'

'Ah ... So what happened ... actually?'

'I can't sleep. I can't do anything. I'm just pacing up and down, going on the internet, arguing with everyone...'

'Mmm ... so what happened?'

Another couple of times around that particular circuit, then 'Got into a bit of trouble.'

Ah.

'How?'

'Irregularities ... shite really...'

'Irregularities ... at work?'

Nods.

'Ah. So what do you do ... at work?'

'Pensions department. I ... run the pensions department...'

Ah.

I had thought that we were on a route to something about internet porn, or sexual harassment, but I'm wrong, as usual.

'They're saying I embezzled ... some funds...'

Ah.

Sometimes, if you assume the worst in what a person is going to say, it gives them permission to confess it – the worst. It can save a lot of time, cuts through a lot of lies.

It *can* be a high risk strategy.

'So what did you steal?'

He looks a little startled. Thinks for a moment.

'I *borrowed* some money. I *actually* paid it all back ... but it was quite a lot...'

Ah. So. Nicking people's pensions. Tricky. 'Why?'

He flashes me a look. I'm needling him. I don't quite know why. I seem to be angry myself this morning. Don't really know why. He shrugs. He seems to collapse in on himself.

'Debts. Online gambling.'

Arse. 'How much?'

Clearly I have pushed him too hard. He looks irritated. 'Are you here to help me or not?'

'I don't know. How do you want me to help you?'

'With my sleep … My *depression*…'

'Do *you* think you're depressed?'

He shrugs, hopelessly. The fight's all gone out of him.

'I'm frightened of going to prison. I'm not *like* that. Do you think I'll go to prison?'

'Depends how much you took. I don't know. I would imagine so.'

He sits looking at the floor. Tears of self pity well up. I fight the urge to feel sorry for him.

'Are you feeling suicidal?'

Shakes his head.

'Drinking too much?'

'Bit.'

'Drugs?'

'*Never!* I would never sink to that!'

I feel this intense, subjective urge to *do something*. I feel this extraordinary urge to make this into a medical problem, to give him a diagnosis. Gambling addiction? Depression? Anxiety? Sociopathic personality disorder with narcissistic traits? I could prescribe him a major tranquiliser for his impulsivity, an anti-depressant for his mood, a benzodiazepine for his anxiety, and psychotherapy for his personality, were that available on the NHS, which it surely isn't.

I feel this need to give him an account of his experience which is somehow different, or more authoritative than the one that he has already given me. To re-describe him as a patient, and grant him all the benefits that that description will bring. It's not because I care that much. I feel angry this morning. I don't know why, but the wells of my compassion are running dry. And I don't think that I would like this man at the best of times. Tired and angry as I am today, this seems to be the only way out of this conversation: to assert a diagnosis, issue a prescription, enact the performance of a complete, diligent medical consultation. You'll see; everyone will be happy with that transaction, no one can possibly object. But to do so would be to collude in a lie. I suppress the urge to lie. It takes some force, but I do it. I manage.

'I can't quite see ... what I can do to help with your situation. Gamblers Anonymous?'

'No point. No cards left to gamble with. Can't gamble in prison. Can't you give me something that will make me feel better? Don't *you* think I'm depressed?'

I think you're ashamed. I think you're feeling guilty. I think you're afraid. I think you've trashed your life and haven't quite acknowledged the fact. I think you've dishonoured yourself. I think that you've given in to the worst of yourself, and can't quite believe what you have become. I think a lot of things, but: 'I don't think the word "depressed" quite covers it.'

'So there's *nothing* that you're going to do to help?'

'Few sleeping tabs? Can't ... quite think of anything else right now...'

'*Fuck*...' Shakes his head, stands all of a sudden, heaves up his burden from the floor, stomps out.

v

A good idea, a good word, according to Plato, 'carves nature at its joints, as a good butcher would.' Some words and ideas in medicine do that deftly. A broken leg, for example, is as clear and accurate a description of a thing in the world that one could wish for. You can even *see* the outlines of the problem there on an x-ray as clear as moonlight shadowed through trees on a dark night: broken/not broken. Whole domains of medicine, domains which are just as real, and just as important as the fixing of broken legs, aren't like that. Depression, for example, isn't like that.

Increasingly, worldwide, diverse classification systems are used to define, and carve up psychiatric illness. This can be helpful, in order to clarify what exactly it is we're talking about when we use a certain word, such as depression. It's invaluable if we are trying to do science – to ascertain whether a treatment or an intervention helps, or harms. These systems can also be used to determine what sorts of things doctors get paid for treating, and, in some systems, for what illnesses and treatments patients will be reimbursed by their insurance companies. One such system, widely used in the US, is called the DSM, or 'Diagnostic and Statistical Manual'. The DSM was created, at least in part, to iron out startling inconsistencies in how different doctors might diagnose and treat patients presenting with the same kinds of complaints. It has an appealingly logical tree and branch struc- ture, which is very similar to how all biological classification systems are organised: family trees. Because in nature, that's how creatures have evolved. Everything is ultimately related; we all share common ancestors.

Criteria for the diagnosis of depression according to the DSM are complex, but involve, amongst other things, the following.

Specific symptoms, at least five of these nine, present nearly every day:

1 Depressed mood or irritable most of the day, nearly every day, as indicated by either subjective report (e.g. feels sad or empty) or observation made by others (e.g. appears tearful).

2 Decreased interest or pleasure in most activities, most of each day.

3 Significant weight change (5%) or change in appetite.

4 Change in sleep: insomnia or hypersomnia.

5 Change in activity: psychomotor agitation or retardation.

6 Fatigue or loss of energy.

7 Guilt/worthlessness: feelings of worthlessness or excessive or inappropriate guilt.

8 Concentration: diminished ability to think or concentrate, or more indecisiveness.

9 Suicidality: thoughts of death or suicide, or has suicide plan.

On one level, this checklist approach to analysing symptoms seems to make a lot of sense. Within its scope lie most people whom you might think of as being very unhappy, or unusually unhappy, or unhappy for a very long time. These are people who conform to whatever it is we mean, when we use the word 'depression'. It seems important that we have the tools to make some kind of distinction between categories of unhappiness – those kinds that merit medical interest, and those that don't – and this list of symptoms makes a good stab at making these kinds of distinctions. The borders might be fuzzy; it's not obvious, for example, why you might require five out of the nine symptoms, and not four, or six, or four and a half, and it's not clear either what you should say to a person who falls just outwith the scope of the tool – but science is like that, most of the time. Instruments are always less precise than we would like, lines have to be drawn, and judgement calls have to be made. Once you have clear diagnostic lines, even somewhat arbitrary ones, you can start thinking clearly about a thing. You can measure it and count it, you can do science on it, including reliable, blinded controlled trials looking at treatments and outcomes, and doctors can start advocating for their patients, using words and ideas which everyone understands.

But there are problems with this approach. That simple symptom list above is festooned with exceptions and conditions. For example, it doesn't count if your symptoms are brief and of recent onset. It doesn't count if they are understandable – a reaction to something bad that has happened, say. It doesn't count if the symptoms are the result of bereavement. Or drug abuse. Or if your guilt is a reasonable response to something really bad that you have done, like embezzlement. Or your all-pervading fear is a reaction to a realistic possibility, like a prison sentence. These other shades of unhappiness are disposed of under different headings and different categories, some overlapping, some on completely different branches, yet each as fuzzy as the other, and each with its own prognostic and therapeutic implications. Anxiety disorder. Sociopathic personality disorder with narcissistic traits. Adjustment disorder. Bereavement. *Just being an arse*. Each but the last has its own place bordered with its own soft lines of demarcation. My man doesn't fall convincingly into any of them.

The effect of a classification system that *looks* biological is to affect the way that we think about it. It is to reify mental illness, to make it into an objective thing in nature (rather like a broken leg) rather than a subjective experience, malleable by culture, history, language, persuasion or preference. Classification systems based on biological genealogy only do the work of describing well if the thing being classified has a stable form in nature, and has evolved through a process of natural selection or descent. It is hard to see how this can be the case for many mental experiences and maladies. To view psychological maladies as families of biologically related illnesses is to risk distorting one's understanding of them.

The history of any culture talking about states of mind, shows culture faithfully reflecting and exploring the currents and preoccupations of its age. It is as if the thing that is being talked about changes its shape with each generation that talks about it. It is as if the words that we use – 'depression', in our epoch – not only describe, but generate, meaning.

We don't know for sure how other people in other times perceived their world, or how the world within themselves felt to them. We don't really know this for sure of others in our own time, either. We can only really know it about ourselves, in fact, and even that can be unreliable. But stories surely help: they tell us *something*, though through a distorting, fogged lens, and descriptions of undifferentiated unhappiness – madness, despair, rage, shame, jealousy and melancholy – appear consistently in all of the history and literature that we have. The despair of Job in the Old Testament, abandoned by a capricious God, or the rage of Achilles in Homer, the fear of Everyman in the plague infested medieval Europe, and the terrible maddening hurt of King Lear at the ingratitude of his daughters – these are all recognisable emotions, although the words, grammar, syntax, and beliefs through which they are experienced and expressed seem alien.

Culture has always viewed the workings of the mind and its dysfunction through the prism of its own world view, and medicine has always been a part of that process. The way medicine thinks about mind changed, profoundly, radically, in the 1950s, and quite by chance. As part of a series of experiments to determine whether a class of compounds derived from coal tar, the phenothiazines, might act as an antimalarial, it was discovered that a subgroup of these, whilst having no anti-microbial effect, altered the behaviour of rats trained to climb ropes, in effect, sedating them, creating loss of interest, or indifference to their surroundings. The discovery of chlorpromazine in 1950, the first effective treatment for schizophrenia, started a revolution in how doctors and their patients thought about mental distress, and initiated a sequence of events which resulted in the possibility of treating unhappiness with drugs. It's difficult to be significantly unhappy in the West now, at least for very long, without being exposed to the various competing ideas of brain chemistry. A vast amount of data has accumulated concerning the biochemical substrates which are involved in creating the mental phenomena of our inner lives, and, until the 1990s at least, a great amount of money was invested in researching the possibility of how drugs might influence these.

The new biochemical science of mind, together with the hierarchical, biological categories of DSM system for classifying psychological symptoms, has given energy to this new idea: that there are specific, distinct and definable mental illnesses with unique, underlying biochemical signatures, and that there are specifically interacting drugs which can pinpoint these illnesses and alleviate the distress that they cause.

This chain of invention and discovery – of psychotropic drugs, biochemistry, biochemical drug 'receptors' – and the evolving biological classification systems for psychological illness, have proceeded jointly, arm in arm, in a fertile, creative interaction, fuelled by money, patient demand, psychological pain, advertising and scientific ideology. It seems, not so much that drug discoveries have created the key to unlock cures for illnesses, but that the keys and the locks have created and defined one another.

This process has been accompanied, in turn, by an enormous increase in the rate of diagnoses of illnesses of the mind. New drugs and new drug receptor sites have greatly increased the range of illnesses that it is possible to have. It isn't clear whether we are happier or unhappier in our lives in the West, despite our huge material wealth, but it certainly seems to be the case that we think and talk about it differently. There has been not so much an explosion of unhappiness, as much as a re-describing of different shades of distress, in terms of medical diagnoses, brain science, biochemistry and drugs. By describing a person as depressed, or describing yourself as such, you aren't simply being given, or accepting, a diagnosis, but buying into an ideology – a wholly new, arbitrary, invented, and perhaps unscientific, world view.

When I experience my inner world, I can't escape the history and culture that shapes it. This modern, biochemical idea of depression is only weakly descriptive of what it signifies, but powerfully generative.

vi

But there *is* something in there – in that inner world – that needs to be described.

Because a thing evades description, and changes within the environment in which it exists, and because it can't be measured or seen but only felt or experienced doesn't make it in any sense less real, or less important. There is something there that matters, that we need to understand and be able to talk about. Compassion urges us to help; we need to know how best to do that. But we can neither talk nor think about the bad thing, nor find ways to fight it, without the right words and the right ideas to do the work for us. There is an urgency about this. We need to get it right.

One cold morning not so very long ago I'm starting a busy morning in my surgery. I notice a message left for me, marked urgent, from Maddie's mum. The message is short and sombre in tone. She and her now-teenaged daughter are away on a break. They are in Florida. She had had a call from work. Her husband hadn't been in for a couple of days. Work were just wondering if he was sick? She'd told them to call the police.

The message is brief, to the point; I know well enough what it is saying.

I don't have time to do anything about it – I have 13 patients to see, I am behind, as always, and I have to keep my head together.

He was in his late forties. He had an unhappy marriage. His wife had left him and taken their daughter. He was drinking. He had stolen money. He was facing a prison sentence, he had told me as much. His daughter didn't want to see him any more and that was just unbearable to him. His wife said she wanted the house and the car, and he *loved* his car. She had come to hate him. I think she was punishing him too, although how could *I* say? He hadn't seen his family for many months. *Why was it not obvious to me then, on that day when I had seen him last, as it was obvious to me now, what it was that he was going to end up doing? Why wasn't I kinder? Why didn't I see what his shame might drive him to?*

A couple of police officers turn up at my surgery just as I am finishing. A young man in his late twenties, clearly anxious, and an even younger female trainee, who is pale and silent throughout. The man takes my name and details, enters them into his handheld device, tells me that they need a doctor to certify a party as deceased, and asks would I help. *Of course I will help, of course.*

It is very cold and I go out without my jacket, and by the time I am in the back of the police car, I am shivering. The two up front are silent. The woman radios ahead to say that we are on our way. They drive me to the grand old house by the loch, about half a mile from my surgery, down a long muddy lane lined by the bones of winter trees. We stop in a pebbled driveway and the police man says, 'Nicest house in town…' but his partner says nothing and the conversation dies. The house is dark, as if it had been shut up.

At the bottom of the long garden, two more police officers are posted. They stand, flat faced in the grey light, looking at their feet. An older plain-clothes guy, in charge, wearing a dark suit, carrying a styrofoam cup, checks his watch, sees me coming and chucks a cigarette butt into the undergrowth by the loch. I realise too late that I have forgotten my gloves.

'Thanks for coming, Doc,' he says, indicating to me a bench, a few metres away, at the water's edge.

'Is it safe?' I ask, like an idiot, and the older police officer purses his lips, says nothing, just indicates with an open hand.

A man, his back to me, sits on a bench at the water's edge on a patch of lawn, surrounded by reeds. It's the middle of winter so there is thin ice on the water, a light mist obscuring the further shore, and frost on the grass which crackles under my feet. He is wearing a business suit. He sits, unmoving, slumped forward like he is feeding the ducks. He has a clear plastic bag on his head, tied with a red silk neck tie, an empty bottle of vodka at his feet and some empty foil pill packets scattered on the frozen mud.

I feel for a pulse on his neck. His skin is cold and solid and scarcely yields to the touch. I open his shirt, push aside a silver St Christopher necklace, and listen for his heart, which is silent. There is cold sweat making his shirt cling to his skin. I think *whose air am I breathing in,* as I loosen the knot, pluck away the plastic bag, and shine a light into the pupils, which are misted over. There is no pupillary response, his head doesn't move on his neck, and he is already stiff with the cold.

They drove me back to my work to give a statement. After, I tried over and over to wash my hands of his sweat.

vii
Half a year has passed, and her son is still haunted by the memory of the man sitting dead on the bench by the loch.

Early August. He has been called back from holiday early because she has deteriorated. She had tried swallowing some tea, and choked on it. Then she panicked. Then, whenever she tried to swallow after that she became frightened, and the fear itself was causing her to choke, so that she was choking and spitting almost all of the time. In another time, or another place, she might have been tube fed at this point, and her pain prolonged indefinitely, but she and her son had discussed this eventuality. She knew what she wanted and what she feared.

One strangely happy afternoon a month or two prior, they had spent an hour sitting in the garden of her old house drinking tea. They had taken off from the nursing home, and impulsively driven to the village where she had lived most of her life, where she had brought up her children, where she had been happiest for longest. It had felt as if she had taken a holiday from her illness. It was early spring and her husband's garden, long neglected now but still beautiful, was alive with birds. She had said, unbidden, 'There's something that I want to talk about.' She sensed that her time was short and wanted its end really. In that happy moment, unburdened and tranquil in one another's company for a change, they had taken the opportunity to have that conversation that comes, eventually, to all parents and their children, or should.

If you had a stroke, what would you want? If you couldn't eat or drink, what would you want? If you couldn't communicate, or couldn't look after yourself, if you were totally dependent, or couldn't breathe or swallow, or if you were in pain that wasn't going to end, what would you want?

It felt like a relief to be clear about these things. It felt like the first adult conversation that they had had for years. As he helped her to her feet to go back inside, he had hugged her spontaneously, for the first time in ages. Almost found it in himself to tell her that he loved her, but didn't quite.

Now she is on a syringe driver, with morphine and a strong sedative, and is powerfully asleep. Her mouth is dry, and she is not distressed – her son thinks that she is not distressed. It is clear to him that she isn't going to wake again, and so he sits, holding her hands. He is trying hard to remember the last good thing that she ever said to him, and then to hold on to it tight. He can't remember the last good thing that she said to him.

She has been deteriorating for many years. It has been a gradual thing. The happier times became fewer, the music and reading less and less and the friendships too – now these friends are reduced to the loyal core, to those who understand properly what she had been to people, and give back a portion of what she has over the years given out. Her son, arm in arm with her through every step in her long decline, has tried his hardest to slow it, but nothing has ever worked. Sometimes she was happy, and sometimes she was sad, and then she was mostly sad. But at some point, a year or two after her husband died, her mind had set, like a jelly. The fluctuations in her mood lessened. She became locked in her grey state. She stopped trying: she stopped reading, or singing, or playing music, then she stopped eating much, and from then on, pretty much, she was always sad.

For years he had tried to persuade her that she was depressed, that she was sick, that this was an illness, that it could be treated! She would accuse him of pestering her. She wasn't depressed! She couldn't be unhappy if she tried! And then if he persisted, she would become angry, and if he persisted more, she would cry, which he hated and which she knew he hated. And then one day she was persuaded by a kind doctor to admit that she *was* depressed. That she had been so for years: her depression had been eating her up, like a grub hatched in her soul. *I feel like I've just come out as homosexual!* she giggled, chirpy and odd, on the way out of the clinic, surging ahead, no need now for a frame, nor her son's arm to lean on. She was started on Prozac, and although the knowledge of this diagnosis and the understanding that this gave her, gave her a kind of clarity – 'depression' being a powerful word – the drug made no difference to her at all.

Perhaps it all came too late, her son thought, as he sat beside her bed, wondering to himself what had been the last good thing that his mother had said to him.

———

You can only spend so much time with an unconscious person: even, especially, with one who isn't going to wake again. Her son needs to come up for air. He stumbles from the darkened room out into the August light.

The situation with his mother and that suicide that he attended, even though months have passed, have put him in a nihilistic frame of mind. Try though he wants, struggle though he might, he can't shake it off. He can't get out of bed in the morning. There is a heft to everything: his limbs drag, his heart is a weight in his chest, the very air he moves through is thickened. But it's warm outside and the sun is shining, and right this moment, just now, he is going out to enjoy the sun. He has decided to take a break. It's only a short walk from where she lies to the beach.

Her breathing is stertorous and shallow, her mouth dry, she is unresponsive, twitching a little, possibly a little opiate toxic.

There is a cool wind from the east, which is a relief. He breathes deeply. The sea air! All the way from the north it comes, from the steppes, the clean pack ice. He walks along the sand on the sea line, dodging the foam, to the old harbour. He has a photo of himself as a baby taken in this very place. It's saved on his computer and flashes up, randomly when he's working; it distracts him. In the photo he is sitting upright in an old, massive sixties pram. He can't be more than five months old. He is squinting into the autumn sun, smiling reflexly at whoever is smiling at him; you can see the shadow of the person taking the photo cast on the grass by the ancient sea wall.

The son is troubled by his own grey mood. Not because he isn't functioning well, and not because he is experiencing any pain, as such. He is in a contemplative frame of mind – he is melancholy, more aware than usual of the dark tones. But he is nonetheless worried about what it all might mean for the future. He is worried about becoming, himself, undefended. He is worried that he, too, is harbouring the grub, that he incubates it too, that it is growing inside *him*, feeding, growing fat. Sometimes he wakes at night thinking that there is a dead man's sweat on his hands, and when he has that thought he has to get up and wash.

He swears under his breath, shakes his head, takes a deep swallow of fresh northern air, says to himself 'Stop it!' He walks the length of the old harbour and back, then makes his way round the headland, passing the ruined castle, the golf courses, and out towards the West Sands, and heads north along the lines of the dunes towards the river estuary.

For years he has taken comfort in this austere thought: that it is the self deceptions that we think sustain us, that are the ultimate source of our unhappiness. You can't begin to live well, to be happy, unless you are honest. You can't accept life, unless you understand it.

So, to chop it all back:
- Everything comes to an end. We all die. In the end, we all lose everything.
- We are alone. There isn't any God.
- Life has no external purpose. There is no external agent to give it meaning.
- And, given that, we are free to make of it what we want.

For her son at least, the pain of existence lessened greatly when he read this, bleak though it might seem – though no one else with whom he has tried to discuss the paradox has seemed much interested.

Thin sheets of shallow water slide over one another like coloured panes of glass, catching the late sun. Far out to sea, lines of oystercatchers fly, dipping in and out behind the breaking surf line. He wishes he could tell his mother about all this natural beauty, because she would have appreciated it, and then he realises that he is already thinking about her as if she were dead, and that he will continue to have this thought, recurring from time to time, for the rest of his life, and that everything about him is changing, changing continually, and always will.

Right now, the question of whether brain chemistry can tell us anything useful about how we should live our lives seems unimportant to him. No one knows whether drugs can *really* make people happier, and how we would know, and what we really mean by 'really' and 'happier'. They seem to sometimes, and maybe that's all that matters. The arguments that he has had over the years with friends and colleagues about Freud, psychotherapy, CBT, mindfulness, meditation, yoga, acupuncture, homeopathy, Reiki healing, all that stuff, whether it works, whether it doesn't, whether it's just a ritual, culture or religion, or whatever, seem like noise just now.

Chop it all back:

Live your own authentic life. Make the best of what you have, of what you've been given: that seems to be what matters. Anything that helps with that, well, good! And anything that detracts from that, takes away from you your capacity to live your best version of life, the best one that you possibly can, is harm.

He still can't remember the last good thing that she said to him, though, before she slept.

It takes half an hour to reach the end of the promontory: a narrow finger of sand, dune and grass that reaches out into the river estuary. The water here is dark and deep and flows hard in currents around the headland, and the wind whips up in a vortex. Stand up straight and look north to where the sandbanks are, and you can see the seals sometimes, dark snouts poking above the chop, tiny whiskered cones on the feathered grey. She had taken them there, to this spot when they were little, held each by the hand and they had stood as straight as soldiers, and she had taught them to sing to the seals. She had taught them that if they angled their mouths in a way to the wind and sang as loud as they could, they would see the seals' heads rising above the waves to hear their calling. He stands as straight as he can and throws his head back and sings a note into the wind; the wind snatches his voice from his mouth, carries it out to sea.

She had said: 'I remember when I was four or five, Jim came to visit, unexpectedly. Everyone was really upset about something. Jim was in a terrible rush, he was looking for something, and was agitated – everyone was angry. Jim was going here and there opening drawers, muttering under his breath, and Dad was saying "Jim!" pleading. And Mum was saying, "I won't have this in my house!" I wanted to help Jim to find whatever it was ... I can't remember what it was ... but they made me go to bed. I couldn't sleep. I could hear them all arguing downstairs. I hate it when people argue, you know that, it just makes me want to cry. Then there was a bang, and it was quiet then for a while. I think Mum and Dad must have gone to bed too, but I still couldn't sleep because I was wondering what it was that Jim had been looking for.

'Then Jim came into my room. He was trying to be quiet, but he seemed disorientated, he kept bumping into things. He said "Joy! There's something I want to show you!" He stood there ... I could see him standing there, swaying in a ribbon of silver light that came through a tear in the blackout. I didn't know what to do, I didn't want to get into trouble, but he said "Come on, Joy! I've got something to show you!" and so I stood up, scuttled over to him with my blanket to stay warm. It was cold, and the fire went out at night in our house. Anyway, he took my hand, put his finger over his mouth and said "Shh!" and we went together out of the flat and down the

steps. My feet were cold, and I tried to tell him, but he just put his finger to his lips and said "Shh", but when we got to the bottom, to the passage to the drying green round the back, it had been raining and the ground was wet, so he crouched down in front of me and said, "Climb aboard the horsey then!", and I could smell something on his breath which I know now was whisky, but I couldn't know that then because no one in my house drank. Isn't memory a funny thing?

'So I climbed onto his shoulders in my nighty with my blanket wrapped around my shoulders and I tugged on his ears and I kicked my heels and said "Giddy up then!" and I remember Jim laughing. He trotted and staggered and whinnied like a horse, all the way down the alley to the drying green, then stopped, holding one of my knees with his hand and pointing with his other finger at the sky, he said, "Look at that, Joy! Look!" And there was an enormous harvest moon rising, just above the roofs of the houses opposite. The biggest, rusty-red full moon that you could imagine. He wanted to show me the moon, as if it were a present. As if it were something that he could give me. Isn't that lovely?'

The Ghost in the Machine

Early January and fiercely cold. It was ten years ago, near enough.

There is a wind whipping in from the North East which has caught you on the ridge; it has had you in its teeth for the last hour, and has slowed you down, and drained you. You hide under a huge stone on the saddle between *An Mealach* and the next step, the steep east face of *An Stac*. You want to rope up, but with gloves off your fingers quickly grow numb and harnesses and knots become hard and stiff, and it's all taking too much time.

'Is this wise?' asks Andrew, who is right to be cautious.

'Yeah!', knowing, of course, that this is by no stretch wise, and that that is why you are there.

The ascent was fine. The snow soft enough to kick steps, yet crisp enough to be a comfort rather than a hazard. The steep sections were rocky enough to offer spikes to loop the rope around, but you didn't need them, no one would slip, and besides, out of the wind, snacked up and with a gulp of tea, you were feeling strong again.

There are times of heightened sensation or strong emotion – love or hatred, sex, fear, exultation, pain – when you are reminded, insistently, of the terms and conditions of your time on the world: that you have this transient possibility of experiencing the world from your own unique, free, personal, perspective; that your time is short; and that you know this. That is, you are aware that you are alive, and that sometime you are going to die. Most of the time you don't think too much about it. In fact, mostly you live life carelessly, as if it is for ever. Sometimes, though, during those heightened times, you are reminded. You see life from that all-embracing perspective, and it is sad and thrilling. You tell yourself that that is why you sometimes do things that seem objectively stupid: things that make you frightened sometimes result in pain, for yourself, for others. It brings you in closer proximity with those terms and conditions. If you believed in her, you would say that it brings you closer to God.

That feeling of being – of being strong, in a rhythm, of walking, then climbing, hand over hand, the thunk of an ice-axe now buried deep in strong supportive pack, moving purposefully upward in an austere and arduous environment – this is a large part of it, why you're here.

It took an hour or so, but at the top, on the flat, icy summit plateau, you were exposed to the wind again and now it's an hour later, and the sun is going down. The plan had been to complete the circuit, traverse to Ben Lawers, then the long descent to where you left the car, at dawn, seven hours ago, but that descent will now take place in darkness. Not dangerous, probably, but very, very long. A few hundred metres below you, lost in a flurry of cloud and ice, is a little lochan where you fished a few summers previously, when it was so hot that you had stripped down to a t-shirt and underwear, caught a little silver trout and threw it back, swam, ate lunch naked on the rocks under the sun, and headed down again. You can't picture what that descent might look like now. Steep on the map, but less than what you have just climbed. You don't fancy it. Unknown territory and the weather is closing in.

So retreat. The ascent had been easier than expected. Pick your way down over the rocks, back to the saddle and the shelter of the big stone, then it's a stroll down to the lochan with its little silver trout. So.

But the descent was awful. Cold, tiredness, hunger: they make you stupid. Those rocks that felt like stepping stones on the ascent are slippery now, tooth-like, and it has grown colder yet, and the snow steps are obliterated. Down climbing on axe and front points is slow and perilous and you are frightened.

You pause. Cold makes you stupid. It's good to think.

Sit by a sharp rock. Use a sling looped round a spike to secure yourself, sit with your back against it, braced. Rope Andrew in, then he climbs down, much faster now, supported by the tight rope. Thirty metres down, he's not out of the woods, but he's not going to fall. Problem half solved.

Now loop the half way point of the rope round the same rock spike, and half-abseil, half climb the 15 metres that the half length of rope gives you. It's not ideal. No amount of optimism disguises the fact that you will be only halfway down, but that's twice as good as where you are now, and besides, this is taking forever.

There is no *good* decision – crises are like that – but doing nothing is definitely the worst. The cold makes you stupid. The fear that's wrapped around your stomach, makes you stupid. You weren't, you realise, much good at this in the first place. Which makes you stupid.

The 15 metre descent is clumsy but okay, but the place it gets you to isn't. It feels very steep. With a good smack, your axe secures you on the ice, but your crampons are a little loose. On the ascent you hadn't even noticed that, but now, in fact, everything depends on everything being solid, and it isn't. Andrew is shouting something from below, which is probably encouragement, maybe a warning, but really you just need to focus. You pull on the rope to free it, but it snags. You pull again, and it snags again. You start to climb up, with a half-formed notion to free the rope by hand, but then change your mind, thinking, correctly, that that is definitely stupid – what, after all, is the value of a rope? You half turn, to free yourself from the rope which is now loose, and then you snag a tooth of your crampon in your gaiters, and stumble, and then you fall.

———

I met this man, years ago. I hardly knew him, but he told me this story:

He'd fought, sort of, very briefly, in Normandy during the war. He had only one arm, the right amputated below the elbow, and I asked him how he had lost it. Some people are sensitive and you dance around these questions. Others, not.

His granddaughter looked at him with a warm, loving look, then at me, and said, 'Watch it, he'll never stop now you've asked him!'

The old guy leaned forward, supporting his weight on his left hand on a stick and said, 'Well…'

He wasn't a particularly educated man, but he had a gift, or perhaps just the gift of a story to tell, but when he told it, it was as if you were there with him.

'… in 1944, the day after the landings, in some part of Northern France, but God alone knows where really … half running, under fire, one of a line of other soldiers, laden with equipment, half running across exposed ground, not afraid. Not because I'm any kind of hero – far from it – but because in that situation, you just aren't afraid…'

He fixes me through his bright blue, watery eyes, tells me his story. It's well practised. He's told this story to three or four generations, his own parents, his sisters, his daughter, his grand-children, and now me.

'… we're running along this muddy lane, all thick under-growth and these French trees on either side, our heads down so they don't get blown off, just going for it, when I hear this terrible bang and see this kind of red flash, and then I realise that I've dropped my rifle, which you realise is about the worst thing you can possibly do, and I'm thinking I can't leave that behind, the company sergeant will cut my balls off – excuse me sir! – so I pick it up with my other hand, that and the *hand that's still holding the rifle*, and I just run until I catch up with the others, and the company sergeant, he sees me and says, "Where've you been, Jock? What's that you've got in your hand?" And then he goes white in the face and just passes out, and I look down, and I pass out too, and it's the end of the war for me! No right arm! Bingo! Just rehab for me after that!'

He makes the international drinking sign with his stump, winks at me, tipping an imaginary pint jar into his mouth from an imaginary right hand. 'Rehab!'

You aren't afraid. No time to be afraid.

Head down and gathering so much speed that there is no question of stopping yourself.

You are aware first of the impact of the hard ice, the way it rattles your bones, before the conscious knowledge that you are falling, fast, head down. That feeling of being a thing-in-the-world, a stone, gathering speed, being airborne, hammering down onto hard ice, preceded any thought, or reflection, or knowledge. But the axe is still looped around your wrist on its cord. Something in you uses that as a rudder, and that swings you around so that you are on your back now, no longer falling head first, but it offers no resistance to your fall, and below you are black rocks livid against the snow, and below them the saddle.

You aren't afraid, everything is happening and changing too fast for fear. Your left foot glances on the rock – *did you try to stop yourself?* – and there is a crack, but whether that was a sound, or some other perception of some huge cracking, opening somewhere else in the vast universe, you just can't say. There was a red flash, and then a kind of silence, and then you are at rest, flat on your back, on the saddle of the hill.

There is nothing of what you might in ordinary speech call 'pain'. You sit up to look around. The world goes black. You faint.

———

This is all recollection. How could it be otherwise? Any account of a mental event is a recollection, and not the event itself. The thing itself is out of reach. And a narrative so constantly recalled in time ceases to be a memory of an event as such, so much as a memory of all of those many other occasions when its traces have been brought back to mind.

I have a patient who was a soldier in Northern Ireland in the early seventies, at the beginning of the Troubles. A gentle man, whose hands shake. A broken, bloated man in his seventies:

he has watery eyes and smoky breath and he always tells me that he's fine when he clearly isn't. Ted has coronary vascular disease and emphysema, and hides – badly – an alcohol problem, which grieved his wife when she was alive. It grieves him that it affected her, but now he is powerless to remedy it, or feels himself so. There are hundreds of men like this, all over. All doctors are familiar with them, though many are not so kind, gentle, restrained, as my man.

He hardly ever talks about what happened, and never in detail.

'...*but when they ask us, we'll never tell them, never tell them...*' as the First World War ditty has it.

His story sounds, in his telling, like a report to a senior officer.

'... about seven in the evening, we're on foot patrol, when these *kids* call us over: a schoolbag's been slung over the bar of a lamp post. It wasn't so notorious, that road, back then ... We weren't meant to help but we thought *what the hell* ... I remember glancing up at the windows of the flats overlooking, whilst Johnie Irvine marched over with a stick to try to hook it off...'

This seems unbearably naïve to me – amateurish almost, but this is now, and that was then, and besides, I wasn't there. I am aware that my mouth is dry, and I'm sweating. I try hard to focus on Ted's story.

'... so Johnie Irvine's standing on his tippie-toes with this long stick trying to get this stupid bag down, shouting "I can't quite reach..."

'There were a few people gathered, but then I see it's like they're sort of *shrinking* back from us, like they know what's about to happen, and I'm about to shout "Johnie...!" when there's this *crack*, and a silence, and someone yells – like it's news – *sniper!* And we have to somehow get Johnie Irvine back, and what's left of his head. I knew the man! But the thing that

I just can't stop going over and over is that there's this *child* watching, with his mum and his auntie, and he's shouting at us, he's *laughing*. He's shouting, "You're a bunch of stupid *cunts* so you are…" Are you okay, Doctor?'

No – not really. I'm sweating too. My heart is racing, my breathing is a little fast. I'm listening to Ted, but in my head, I am head down, gathering speed, feeling the impact of that hard ice on my shoulders and back; I can see those black rocks rushing by, outcrops from the snow and ice, I'm waiting for that crack, that red flash. I'm having a flashback.

I have a patient, a young man, broken by a car smash he was in a few years ago. He was unscathed, but the girl in the passenger seat, his girlfriend, was killed. His story has that same quality: unadorned, matter of fact, devoid of any sense of self dramatisation.

'… The thing was, I was going too fast. We were going to a party in Jedburgh. You know the little road near St Boswells, near where it crosses the A68? We were late, and I was going too fast and this lorry doesn't see us, and pulls out from a side road, so I swerved… Are you alright, Doctor?'

No – not really.

In the process of the recollection of an event, you give the event meaning. For my soldier, I suspect, because he has told me, the meaning concerns a foul-mouthed child, whom he is ostensibly there to protect, laughing at him as he recovers the remains of his friend from the roadside. *I knew that man!* For the young driver, the meaning is his shame, his guilt, his sense of responsibility, which will never leave him.

In his book, *Achilles In Vietnam*, the American psychiatrist Jonathan Shay describes post-traumatic stress disorder (PTSD) as a condition determined not so much by the intensity of the trauma a victim experiences, as the structure of meaning that he builds around it afterwards. A victim of post-traumatic stress disorder characteristically experiences intrusive flashbacks – waking nightmares – which almost anything can provoke and in which they viscerally re-experience the events of their trauma. The victim of PTSD is hypervigilant, has hair-trigger reflexes which precipitate a physical and mental re-experiencing of the traumatic event. It seems that almost any unrelated thing can kick off their shaking, their mood swings, their propensity to violence. They will often feel intense guilt and shame, and be subject to impulsive rage or remorse, anxiety or depression, and will often self-medicate with alcohol or other drugs.

According to Shay, victims of PTSD often see their trauma in the context of a more generally disordered moral universe, and that it is the nature of the moral context of the injury which will often predict who will survive psychologically intact, and who won't. He uses the hero Achilles as his prototype example. Betrayed by his leader, Agamemnon, who has stolen his slave girl, Achilles sulks in his tent and refuses to fight. The Greeks are threatened by the Trojans, who are burning the Greek invaders' ships and cutting off the possibility of retreat, and so Achilles agrees that his friend and cousin, Patroclus, will fight in his place, wearing his armour. Patroclus is killed and his body dishonoured. Achilles, visited by a kind of shameful madness, goes on the rampage – goes *berserk*, as Shay puts it. He slaughters his Trojan enemies, piles up their bodies in the river Scamander, until it goes red and the river spirits hide their faces for the shame of what has been done to pollute their water. But nothing can expiate Achilles's guilt and shame.

The person who becomes a victim of PTSD might think that they shouldn't have been there in the first place. That they weren't wanted, or weren't competent. That the wrong person died. That their mission was vain, pointless or wrong. That no one who should have done, cared about them, or their welfare. They might think that it was their own selfishness, stupidity, or inaction that caused the event. Or that they were rendered powerless, or had no agency or ability to control what was happening to them. Or that what happened to them was, somehow, shameful.

I didn't have PTSD, or anything like it. Just the ghost of it – a short haunting – and then it went away. Just enough perhaps to understand what people mean when they talk about intrusive thoughts, or flashbacks. I'm not a soldier, I've never fought in war, or had my friend killed in front of me. No one has died by my culpable intention, or my carelessness, pride, stupidity or haste. Not so much that's bad has happened to me, really. But I *was* somewhere where I shouldn't have been. Vainglorious, I made bad decisions, I wasn't prepared, and should have known better. I might have died, but what's worse, so might others. At least that's the *meaning* that I have given it.

But all those successive waves of interpretation were in the future.

You cautiously sit up again, surveying your new world, how it all looked then. It isn't dark, but the sun is lower, and the wind is getting up. It shrieks around your ears. But you came to rest in the lee of the hill, and so are protected a little from the worst of the cold.

You are oddly euphoric. Andrew isn't. He, who has seen everything, who has rushed over, traversing a steep ice field to find you, and has expected to find you dead, is lost for words.

He has had time to think about everything, all the implications, from the moment that he shouted up his warning to you, when you were casting around in a mess of ropes and knots faffing like an old man looking for loose change in a grocer's queue, to the long gathering slide, head down in a tangle of rope, as he saw you disappear behind the lee of a rock. He has heard nothing since, though he has shouted.

'Are you alright?' Worryingly, he is shivering with cold. You, however, are okay. More than okay. Euphoric. Nonetheless, putting to one side for a moment the crack, the red flash, the faint, the left lower leg which doesn't seem altogether *attached*, you really need to get going. Although feeling in this instant god-like, reason tells you that the biochemical whatever-it-is that's going on in your head, whatever it is that's making you feel this way, this *rush*, isn't going to last. You need to get going.

You make to stand. Your intention is never translated beyond that: you may have had an *intention* to stand, but in that instant of intending, you stop. You experience this overwhelming, externally perceived imperative to *not move*. You are yet to perceive anything that in ordinary speech might be called 'pain'.

You once thought that you knew something about all this. You used to have a spider diagram in your head, a web of interconnecting boxes and lines documenting the complex model for how you, and the neurophysiologists who taught you, understood pain.

So, you knew that there were nerves for the fast transmission of pain – nerves that would ring out like fire alarms if, for example, the tough lining of a bone, the periosteum, were breached. There were other nerves for slow pain – the intolerable low level throb of under-treated post operative pain, for example, or the gnawing pain in the pit of the stomach from cancer. There were other lines, the reticular formation, that radiated to the ancient pre-lizard parts of the brain that determine our crudest jellyfish responses to noxious stimulus, things like arousal, sleep, motivation, mood. And others going to the neocortex, the human-person part, which attributes things to pain like meaning, and thence understanding, reasoning, knowledge. There are boxes relating to memory, and boxes relating to emotion (a *huge* box for emotion). There are gates to inhibit pain, and repress it, others to distract from it, or enhance it. There's a box for hallucination and hypnosis, to imagine that you have *no pain whatsoever* or imagine that you do. There are connections to enable us to learn from pain, and others to help us forget. There's a sea of hormones and corticosteroids whose abundance or dearth modulate all of our human responses, and even a quirky back door connection that allows for the possibility of *enjoying* it all. You used to think that these little boxes and their coloured connecting lines just about had it covered. A person with time, brains and money enough could just about construct a pain machine, from your constantly adapting model, with all its lines and coloured boxes.

But *you* have yet to feel anything that in ordinary speech might be called pain. You sit down again, focused entirely on the lower half of your left leg. You have no control. It is as if your leg has *told you* not even to try it. You have as little agency in this new world-of-pain as an archaic jellyfish, washing around in its warm prehistoric sea. You are, for a moment, a thing quite detached from the body that moves you. You are a ghost in the machine.

'You need to try to stand…'
   'I can't possibly stand.'

All day you have been alone; now at the day's end, you have company. A young woman and her man, a soldier on leave, reassuringly helmeted, stop. They didn't have to stop. They have tea to spare, and they shared it, and their life-saving survival bag. With the bag wrapped around you, and, hands shaking, drinking warm tea, you feel for the first time cold. Their generosity threatens to unlock something in you like tears: there's a bottomless pool of tears there, and you're sliding into it fast, you suddenly realise, and you put the brakes on that one hard. *There's a box for emotion, and a box for the repression of emotion.* But you have started to shake now, and the shaking, which you can't stop, brings intimations of pain. Your left leg, now, in some way, some way off from the rest of you, is worryingly numb. You want to keep it that way. When the soldier makes to take your boot off, to try to give your foot some protection, some warmth, you say, 'Ah, ah' and shake your head. *No one is going to move that foot.* The soldier looks grim, shakes his head.

   'We all need to get off this hill.' He pulls out a mobile phone, quarters the ground for a signal.

   Thank God for soldiers, I say.

A few years later Andrew and I were walking on the hills south of Edinburgh. It was January, and, again, cold. We met a small group of people, a worried knot, sheltering in the lee of the wind. One of them, a woman in early middle age, was sat, cold and worried, shaking her head, laughing, saying, 'You all go on, I'll be fine…'

She had slipped and broken her ankle. It's easily done, even if you're the most sensible person in the world. There was no mobile phone reception. Unlike some I could name (*me*), *she* wasn't making a big fuss about it.

Fit again, I jogged down the town side of the hill until I had a bar on my phone, and called for help. Having learned a thing or two over the years, we had a bivvy bag and some tea, which we shared, while she waited for the emergency people, who made their way slowly up the hillside in a buggy with caterpillar treads. We reassured her powerfully, the emergency people and me, held her leg and foot stable while we slipped off her boot, warmed her, checked her circulation.

'It's gas and air…' I said. 'It helps with any pain when we move you. It takes a couple of minutes to work, but it's really good.'

'I had some when I had my two sons. It's really good…'

'There you go: breathe deeply…'

We coordinated her lifting onto the back of the buggy, and wrapped her exposed foot in as many spare socks as we had. She and her friends thanked us: 'You didn't have to do all of that. You didn't even have to stop, we were fine! But thank you!'

I thanked them back, with a degree of emotion that the circumstances didn't really warrant.

My left ankle by now was throbbing, swollen, really quite painful, and it would take me an hour or two to hobble off the hill, and a few days to recover from that. It was like that for years after the accident – the least exertion would give pain, swelling, a limp. It gets me like that still, after a long run, or a day on the hills. In its way it is a pleasant kind of pain. A pleasant reminder of strength regained, returning from somewhere bad; and that injury, that provocation sustained from the exertion of running down that hill over tussocky grass, running back up again to the woman with her fractured ankle, felt heroic. What a good injury! What a good pain! How symbolic it was of recovery! There was more saving that day for me, than for the woman we helped.

———————

It takes, perhaps, 40 minutes for a helicopter to appear.

It's going to be dark soon. Forty minutes of sitting there, even wrapped in the bag, and you have become indifferent: cold, drowsy, immobile. Part of you wishes the others would leave. They are filled with activity and energy and effort and won't stop still for a moment, and it's really tiresome. The soldier and his companion have laid out a great cross of bags and brightly coloured goretex on the plateau nearby, while Andrew is else-where, nursing a patch of mobile phone reception, acting as comms man for the mountain rescue. A couple of other groups of walkers have passed by now, looked darkly at you, shaken their heads, agreed that there was nothing more that they could do, and hurried off into the gathering twilight. Rule number one for emergencies: don't add yourself to the casualty list.

You can tell by the urgency of people's actions, by the serious-ness of their faces and the false jocularity that they use in your presence, that there is a great deal of fear around. There is a great deal of fear around, a great deal of activity, of doing things, for their own sake. Hunched like a beast behind the darkening crags is pain, with his claws and unblinking red eyes, waiting, and beyond him, silent, something quite unknowable, but to you none of that matters now. You are half detached from the world already, huddled and indifferent, chasing after that last remnant of warmth in your core, focused on stillness, not moving, journeying deeper and deeper within.

———

'When you die,' I have said, on countless occasions, to people facing the imminent reality of that, who have wanted to know, 'you disappear gradually into yourself. You go on a journey into yourself. At first you will be aware of the world around you, and the people around you, but it all becomes progressively less vivid, and it all comes to matter less, or matter less immediately. Their presence may be a comfort, especially at first, but they are a long way off, and diminishing, and your own world starts to shrink down too. Any discomfort you may have will diminish too, and you will stop feeling hungry or thirsty, and you will become more and more sleepy, so that you are hardly awake at all. It's like you disappear to a pinpoint, and then you disappear altogether.'

I've seen a lot of people die, and I think that that's what it's like. That's what it feels like. All speculation, of course. The one thing in the world that no one knows. The one question that can't be answered honestly. And that most pressing of questions, too. All speculation, of course. But less so for me now, perhaps, than it might have been before.

———

The rescue guy woke you up quickly though, woke you good and proper.

An orange RAF helicopter arrives, wobbling in the sky, buffeted by the high wind, then flies off again worryingly. The engine sound drifts off to nothing, then it returns, a couple of minutes later, finding some wind shadow, a hundred yards off, and then again a little closer. It throws down a line with a man in a bright red jump suit, who lands on the ice, who whacks the ground with two hand axes and crampons, and spiders across followed by two bags of gear on another line. He assesses the situation rather rapidly. Great shadows now growing in the valleys, the grey sky dark, there is perhaps 20 minutes of light enough to function by.

'The boot's coming off.' He concludes. 'Leg's broken. Need to splint it, and get you off.'

You don't have time to say 'No. Fuck off.'

There is never, at any point, any question of *consent*. There's no asking what you want, what you feel.

'Breathe on this.'

Hands a battered face mask attached to some kind of cylinder.

'It's gas and air. It's used in child-birth...'

'... I know...' you say, breathing deeply, while he rapidly undoes the boot, slips it off, assesses the damage, sucks air in between his teeth, but you are lost for an instant in that red world of pain and blackness. You faint again, wake, breathe as hard and deep and fast on the cylinder as you can.

'It's empty!' you say.

How many times in the delivery room, have you heard a labouring woman say that? 'The cylinder's empty!' and you have reassured her without really checking, because in real life the cylinder's never empty?

'It's not empty. You've got some kind of fracture-dislocation and your foot's a bit blue and there's no pulse, so I'm going to pull on your foot and put a splint on it. You might want some more of that gas first...,' he says, pulling a brightly coloured emergency splint from his kit bag.

You try to find the words *'Are you fuck...!'* and 'There's no gas in the cylinder', but have no time to assemble the relevant concepts because the soldier is grasping your thigh and the rescue guy is cradling your foot and saying, 'On the count of three...' You are sucking as hard as you can on the empty cylinder, enough to make you dizzy, and then you hear someone screaming out, and you disappear again into the red world of pain, and then the world goes black, and then you wake again having been sick in the snow, and your left leg is now encased in a large splint, and you're thinking *that wasn't so bad* ... then *I need to pee...* and rescue guy says, 'Not a chance...'

———

Using memory, I can find and assemble all of the details. The vivid *red* nature of the pain. The fainting. The fear. The shame and guilt subsequently constructed around it all. The anticipation of pain: that distant warning, which froze me to the ice, and almost cost me my life. The sound of a voice, crying out, and that strange detachment from the world, the drifting away, and my indifference and distance, which I wonder now, and wondered at the time, might be what the approach of death is like.

Using memory, I can assemble the vivid representation of all of these experiences, as if they were coloured boxes connected with lines of meaning. It was me: I was there, it was me that was hunched, indifferent, in the belly of that pain. But now is now, and that was then, and all is changed, and the person remembering it all is no more the person who experiences, than the medical student all those years ago, assembling the coloured boxes and lines and thinking *that means pain,* understood pain. The memory of pain is no more than its representation. It isn't *pain.*

———

He works fast. The able bodied are winched off first, then you and he in a shared harness, you cradling the gas canister because there is swinging and bumping as you are hoisted aloft, and the snowy world spins around on its new axis, then more swinging and bumping as you cross the lip of the helicopter and are deposited in its belly, which is half an inch deep in ice and water, and smells of feet. Rescue Guy stows his gear and throws your gas cylinder into the corner, shouts 'It's bloody empty!' at his mate, the winchman, who shrugs his shoulders and points skyward, and the helicopter gathers its strength, roars in its deep voice and leaps into the sky.

Empty or not, the gas cylinder did its job. You remember everything about that rescue. The fall, the fear, the crack, the red flash, the faint, the vomit, the latent pain, the frozen immobility, the slow slide to warm sleep and death, the reassurance of sucking on the empty cylinder, the way it made you dizzy, the reduction of the fracture, done so fast with so little faff, then the spinning, snowy world: you remember it all, but you don't remember any pain, as such.

Rescue Guy's name is Andy. You shake his hand, over-express your gratitude, gushy and drunk by then on the *real* gas that the ambulancemen provided. You thank him for saving your life; you embarrass him.

———

Pain is the word that surely everyone understands; the word whose meaning is clear without pausing for reflection. You know when you have it, and it's incorrigible in its nature. When you have it, no one can tell you that you don't. Its nature lies in its meaning.

The other week a man came to see me. Sombre and grey, he slumped in his chair and told me that he had a pain. '*Here*,' he gestured to the pit of his stomach, fingers and thumb meeting at their tips, cupped hand, the Italian 'tastes good!' gesture, but directed not at the lips but at the epigastrium (upper abdomen). He looked with his watery eyes straight into mine, hunched slightly forwards, eyes clouded with fear. He is 64 and the whites of his eyes are yellowish. Once plump, his skin now hangs off him like an old mac.

You can tell a lot from the hand gesture about the origin of a person's pain. The fist clenched on the breast bone is heart. The thumb run in a line down the arm or the leg is nerve pain. A flat hand on the front of the chest, heartburn. The weeping child with a flat hand clamped to the side of the ear, earache. The tented fingers over the pit of a hunched stomach is pancreas.

'It's there all the time. Started from nothing over the last couple of weeks. Gnawing away in the background. It's nothing much, I hardly feel it, but it's always there. Wakes me at night…' *Fills me with dread* say the lines on his face.

He looks at me with wide open eyes as I examine his stomach, feel for his liver, his gall bladder. There's nothing much to find apart from the hint of jaundice, but he is unsurprised when I order an urgent scan, and unsurprised when I call him in a few days later to share the results with him.

'There's a swelling at the head of the pancreas. It's block-ing the flow of bile. There are some worrying areas in the liver too...'

Pause. Maybe a tear or two, maybe a deepening of the shadow in the lines of that face, a grey look, a confirmation, but no surprise.

'That sounds ... bad.'

'I'm afraid it is ... bad.'

'So...'

I take some blood, write a letter, and do what needs to be done, and then ask him again about his pain, and he seems a little surprised that I have even raised the subject.

'It's fine. The pain's nothing...'

It's just what that pain means.

Drunk on opiates and gas, do you remember how euphoric you were? How totally inappropriate? You might have been sing-ing as they wheeled you into the resuscitation suite. You try to forget that bit, but you can't. Normally a little fastidious about such things, you may have been a little lascivious with the female nursing staff. May have made the odd 'off colour' comment, which you try not to think about too much. Having gored your-self in the groin with your ice axe, you do clearly remember giving the junior doctor helpful advice on her placing of the stitches and her tying of the knots: that recollection punches through, makes you cringe.

You remember that when they took the emergency splint off to take the x-ray, the now inadequately supported fracture hurt like hell, real pain, proper pain, but it didn't matter. Whacked out on fentanyl, you remember recognising this well-attested phenomenon: that though the pain was intense, nuanced, detailed, entirely felt, you were, nonetheless, entirely indifferent to it. It no longer mattered: it was a curiosity. This is how opiates work: they don't take away the pain, they render you indifferent to it. Which tells you something important: in this context at least, the nature of pain lies not in sensation, but in the anguish that it brings.

There's a *huge* box for emotion.

'It's not possible to identify any common factor present in every sensation that we might ordinarily call pain. There's no necessary or sufficient component for a feeling to count as pain. And yet it is a word that *everyone* understands. Its meaning lies in its use – it's an understanding shared by the community of all beings that are capable of experiencing pain, yet inexplicable to any being lying outside that community. For a being *outside* that community, to talk about pain is to talk about the wiring in a fuse-box and wonder what it's like to be electricity.'

I am sitting in a huge, high roofed office in the nicest part of Glasgow, talking to a man I have taken an instant liking to. This is how the world *ought* to be, I maintain: that there should be philosophers with open minds and big offices with views north to Ben Lomond, with threadbare carpets on the floor and a long wall given over to books about *The Phenomenology of Awareness* and a six-inch wide volume of *Kant: A Primer*. The world ought, I believe, to be arranged just like this: that a doctor troubled by a nagging sense that there is something incoherent or incomplete about our ordinary account of pain should email an expert on the philosophy of the subject, and he will meet you in his office, and with all the time in the world, talk with you for a couple of hours as he stands at his white-board and draws boxes with coloured connecting lines, seeking to explain everything that we think we know and understand about suffering, and in the attempt, demonstrate that, with all this knowledge of how it works, we still can't explain what in nature it *is*. That the philosopher will demonstrate to you the truth of your intuition that what everyone in the world thinks they know to be as hard a fact as the table you're sitting at is, by its nature, unknowable.

And then you go for lunch.

'The boxes and coloured lines might tell something about the mechanics of a *felt* pain in the instant of its perception, and that's interesting. But to capture the essence of a sensation like pain, and then to talk about it, we're looking through the lens of memory. We have no access to the thing itself, and the act of looking and remembering always takes place within a context, which always qualifies the nature of the experience we're recollecting. And … well … is there any such thing as an *unremembered* pain?'

———

The doctor in the resus. room looked at the x-ray on the light board, shook his head, gravely. Defensive though you may have felt about the quality and skill of Andy the rescuer's wild-side reduction of your fracture, you can see nonetheless from where you're lying propped up that the crook in your ankle is astonishing. People are gathered around the screen saying, 'Will you look at that!' which is always a bad sign.

'You see,' says the doctor in greens, 'Rescue Guy restored the circulation and saved your foot, but here in the warmth and light, we can do much better than that. The orthopods can hammer it together properly in the morning, but right now I need to pull on it again, straighten it out, or you'll never get a decent return to function, okay?'

He's already limbering up. A slight, good-looking chap, who nonetheless looks about 12, he can't quite contain his anticipation and delight at the prospect of pulling really hard on a foot.

Back in the days before doctors had to be trained in something before doing it, *you* used to be just like that – *admit it*! You *lived* for heroic doctoring, the spatter of blood on theatre greens, but not any more. Now you're a GP. Yet despite not now being of their tribe, you have a sneaking regard for doctors still at the sharp end of medicine: the ones who make instant, rapid, life or death decisions, which would paralyse you; the ones who stick in chest drains, and crack open chests, call urgently for six units of whole blood, stat!; the doctors who get to charge the defibrillators and shout 'stand clear!' and 'shock!' Doctors who, unlike you, don't overthink everything.

He says to someone, over his shoulder, the charge nurse probably, who's needing the bay for someone else, 'Just a sec. I just need to pull on this foot...' and then approaches with a fake, reassuring smile. Again, you try to say *No! Definitely not!* but haven't quite the time to find the words. Brandished like a quill between two fingers, he has a 2ml syringe which he holds up to the light, squirts out an air bubble in that way that they do, and says as he locates the syringe on the

cannula in the back of your hand, 'I'm giving you a little …
midazolam – it'll wo k in an inst t, and you won't remem a
thing abou…'

And that's the strangest thing: despite the absolutely vivid recollection that you have, of the resus room, the crooked bones on the
x-ray, the gung-ho and ethically illiterate young doctor whom,
to this day, you revere, the memory of his (presumably) pulling as hard as he could to straighten, again, your Maisonneuve
spiral fracture dislocation of the fibula, ankle and interosseous
membrane, the actual moment of brutal pulling has been snipped
out and the hour or so that followed too. You would have been
awake: you know this about the drug. He didn't knock you out –
it's not a painkiller; you would have howled like a dog – but
he just snipped out that little bit of life that you wouldn't want,
that *no one* would want. And where in the world *is* it now? That
snippet? That offcut?

So from the perspective of *now*, with respect to *then*, no: there
is no such thing in the world as an unremembered pain, for you,
at least.

Esther is in the early stages of a slow-burn dementia. I have
known her for years and years, she seems scarcely to change.
She is one of my immortals. Unchanging. All doctors have
them, their senile gods and goddesses. She hops and skips down
the corridor like a little bird, perches on the chair in front of
me, takes out a list, and says, 'Doctor, I've got the memory
of a *hen*!' and smiles, and chitters on about her pain: the pain
in her back, the pain in her knees, the pain in her shoulders,
all of the time restlessly skipping from subject to subject, from

body part to body part. Esther is sunny. Despite the repetitive and tedious nature of her conversation, which I realised was the same with everyone not just her doctor, I liked her. Wanting to help her – that being my job – I used to give her painkillers. I instructed her in exercises for her mobility and got physios to see her in her house to prevent her from falling; they prescribed her walking aids which she used to hang her laundry from, and her husband was instructed in the rubbing in of anti-inflammatory gels which he did, on call for 24 hours a day, to soothe her aching limbs until the day that he died, but none of it worked at all. And with every escalation of the painkillers, Esther would grow more wobbly and forgetful and miserable, and she would look tired and grey and old as she said, 'Doctor, I've got the memory of a *hen*,' and tell me about the pains in her back, her knees, her shoulders. And distressed to see her so cast down, I would stop everything, all the painkillers, and she would brighten up again, grow young before my very eyes, the hopping, twiggy, little bird.

Whenever I was away, or distracted by other patients, and Esther saw another doctor, the cycle would be repeated – it's very hard to deny analgesia to a person saying they're in pain – and Esther would grow old and depressed again, until the drugs once again were stopped, and again she would perk up. She always hopped around like that, restless as a sparrow. The thing was, though, she never *looked* as if she was in any pain at all. I don't *know*, because no one could ever know, but I think that Esther's is just a performance of pain. Old, inflexible, stuck in very few, very narrow furrows, I think that it's what her brain *does* now. It does a performance of pain.

'Assuming she's sincere, and assuming that you're not just somehow wrong, then perhaps she's just mistaken? Perhaps she just *thinks* she's in pain, but really she's not?'

The philosopher smiles, as the implications of his question sink in. I can't tell whether he's being serious or not, but the question seems important. I thought that that's the whole point about it: pain isn't something you can be wrong about.

I say to him: 'I want to write about how complex pain is. I want to express exactly what we have been discussing: that pain doesn't have to be bad, it doesn't have to be even felt, it can be forgotten, or never even known about. I want to write about its meaning, and how that meaning changes with every recollection. I want to write about fear, about the placebo effect, the effect of opiates, and the influence that doctors can have on how pain is perceived. I want to write about culture and the performative element of pain, and I want to say something about how well pain illustrates problems in the philosophy of language and mind. I want to write about all of these things. But I'm not doing it just for interest: you see, I think that it *really* matters, in an immediate and practical kind of way. I think we doctors get pain terribly wrong sometimes, and our mistakes arise because of something to do with how we misunderstand it. So I'm planning to write an autobiography of pain, to try to explore it subjectively. But to try to get some distance on it, I'm going to write in the second person. I'm going to start by *addressing myself* – make it about a fictional 'you', who is remembering the details of an accident, which was traumatic and painful at the time, but had no ill effects. I want to use that 'you' as a kind of vehicle for exploring the subject (me) and the objects of his perceptions and memories. What do you think?'

'About the literary device? Why not just write about pain?'

Pause.
'I have this theory...'

I have this theory. I think it all works something like this:

I think that our consciousness is constructed according to certain grammatical constraints, rather like language. I think that a most fundamental grammatical constraint of language *and* consciousness is that of subject and object. In order to be able to think, we need to perceive *ourselves* to be divided from our *perceptions*, the whole inner world divided into subjects and objects, i.e. that we have a pervasive sense of a subjective 'I', a self, a ghost, that perceives objects in the world through sensation, which we then interpret as external (a table, for example) or internal (a pain, say). Or a subjective 'I' that then remembers things, or an 'I' that then thinks things, or an 'I' that then goes off and does things.

Perhaps this subject/object distinction is just a compelling, vivid artefact of our internal grammar. Perhaps this grammatical form is simply a convenience. I think that, in the instant of feeling, or perceiving, remembering, thinking, or doing, that instantaneous and ephemeral state is what we are: we *are* the pain, or the thought, the colour, the sound, the memory, the perception, the action. There is no subjective 'I' that can be independent of its perceptions and interactions. And *then* we remember. And then an infinite number of beads of perception string themselves on this thread of memory, and make us then the complex, continuous, hurting, loving things we call selves.

'Perhaps...'

But I can't really tell whether he thinks my theory stinks and he is just being polite. Our conversation has gone on perhaps a little long. He has been generous with his time. We finish lunch.

'I've loved this conversation,' I say, meaning it.

We say goodbye, intending to meet again, really thrash this one out, and I hope that we do. I'm late for my train. I rush across the Kelvinbridge as the rain comes down; I half run, half hobble down the steps to the metro. My foot aches. It's not unpleasant.

Opiates are the Opiate
of the People: Part 2

'... but Annie's better now. She had a hard enough time at first, just after the separation, but she's resilient. She's coped far better than we'd thought, and it's been *amicable* you know? My husband Paul still gets on fine with Juan, and wee Kira's a gem! That's a positive, we're close by enough ... we can help out. You don't stop caring for them just because they've left home and got married ... that's just when it all kicks off! You don't know *that* when they're tiny, do you? How old are yours now, Doctor? I can remember when they were at school, but they're probably off on their own by now eh?'

That was the flavour of the kinds of conversations we had. Mrs Connely wears trainers and jogging slacks. She is 62, a retired art teacher. She lights the room with her energy: a fidgety energetic woman, always on the move, jiggling with all of the things she still has to do. She is a young, vital 62.

She's clutching at her prescription – HRT – in her right hand, her sunglasses in her left. She's chatting away about her grand-daughter, halfway to the door on her way to the gym, when, suddenly, as if struck by something, some passing thought, she halts, starts to say something, hesitates, pauses, then starts again, says: '*By the way*, Doctor, I've been meaning to mention…'

I've known her for the best part of a decade. I diagnosed her husband, Paul, with the first presentation of his angina shortly after I'd joined the practice. Not hard. He's a few years older, a retired lawyer and still slightly intimidating in his lawyer's way. Despite that he is flourishing and free in his later life, with his tennis and his hill-walking trips with his many old friends. He'd just stopped smoking. He'd looked almost insulted when he'd told me about his symptoms, his fist clenched to the centre of his chest. 'Been about six weeks. Noticed it first when I was out jogging. Now it happens whenever I'm out of breath, but mainly when it's cold. It's not even a pain, more just a sense of dread – *timor mortis*: you feel it, here…,' he knocks twice, tapping on his hollow chest like it's a door, '… and here,' waving at his throat, his jaw, at this thing that grips and suffocates him. That easily-made diagnosis created a bond between us, this couple and me, and now they come to see me for everything, as does their daughter, and now grandchild Kira, who's five. Trust is a privilege. Earned, as they say, and easy to lose.

Their daughter was quite suicidal when her husband left her. It was, or so Annie thought, entirely her own fault. She had done this *stupid, impulsive thing* one weekend when her husband was away filming in China. Annie is an artist too, like her mother, perhaps more talented, though less rooted. She had a hellish adolescence, ricocheting between partners and pills, new starts and half-completed college courses, but those last few years have been calmer, with a studio in Leith paid by her father. She had her husband Juan, a home, and now the baby. Calmer that is, until she fucked it up with this *stupid and impulsive thing*. Only it wasn't really *that* impulsive: Kira was staying with her other grandparents that weekend, and some rebel part of Annie had clearly planned the whole damned thing, and, though he had tried to, Juan couldn't get beyond that – the fact that she had *planned* it.

Annie, pacing, fidgeting, in that same space where her mother stands before me now, was saying: 'The thing is, I still *love* him, and he loves me...' Annie's restlessness, though reminiscent of her mother, has nothing of her mother's joy in life; Annie's is all self-blame and self-hatred. *I* think that Juan is a prig and needs to get over himself. I have no time for Juan's grand Iberian jealousies, his operatic emotions. He is my patient too, but I can't, I confess, like him as I like the others. I find I tire of him going on and on about his wife's Facebook love affair. I find I can't not take sides. Vainglorious Juan, I think, could save himself and his daughter and the whole of his little world a whole lot of pain if he could just find it in his heart to forgive. But that's *my* privilege: that of being disinterested, a witness. And of course I say nothing to Juan as he rants, nor Annie as she paces, as she clutches a handkerchief to her mouth, whilst Kira, then three, wraps herself around her mother's thigh. Her mother wails: 'How could I have been so stupid? So selfish?'

Blind to their daughter's complex self, Mrs Connely and her husband don't know anything of any of this. They see Annie as a blameless victim and her husband's decision to leave his wife, their daughter, and their granddaughter, as inexplicable. At times Mrs Connely has been so angry, she just can't bring herself to speak to her son-in-law. Communication takes place through Paul. His lawyer's training comes in handy here. All of this, of course, adds to Annie's distress. Few things being worse, for an essentially good person, than to be taken for blameless, when everything is, obviously, in fact, *all your fault*.

And all of this back story is crammed in somewhere at the back of my head when Mrs Connely pauses, a hand on my door, a cloud crossing her clear, sunny, face, and says, '*By the way*, Doctor, I've been meaning to mention something...'

By the way. By the way.

———

In my last year of school, I shared with my best friend the main role in our school's production of *Everyman*. We did alternate nights, Niall and I: his performance was the more reliable, his grasp of the lines more solid, and in the end he became the preferred of the two of us in the show, which we toured in local churches. I suppressed my envy, which I felt keenly at the time, and it didn't affect our friendship, though we have lost touch now. But I like to think still that the best of my performances equalled the best of his, and mine had the more disruptive passion.

Everyman is a medieval mystery play. It's set in a world just post bubonic plague, and it's about life, sex, friendship, remorse, sin, redemption and the inexplicably abrupt intervention of death. We were 16. We created this scene: Everyman lolls with his mistress and friends, drunk, on a raised wooden dais set centre stage, dances to soft music, wriggles and paws at her bodice, sups on wine. I don't imagine for a second that it was much good at all, but we put everything into that show. As happens at that stage in life, there had been a few deaths among our age group: a boy in the year below, swimming with his friend in the Tay, had drowned; another, bought a motorbike by his parents for his 18th, had driven it at speed into the back of a truck and died that death.

After the show, we, the cast, and some of our younger teachers, would sit on the beach and drink and smoke and watch the stars in the sky, and there would be wriggling in and out of towels and swimming gear, the supping of wine, and some pawing too. That was what the late seventies were like.

In the scene we created, Everyman stands, yawns, stretches, staggers a little, and drunkenly bids his friends farewell. As he is walking away from the tableau, a voice, the voice of Death, but hideously amplified, rasps: 'Everyman stand still! Where goest thou so merrily? Hast thou thy maker forgot?' And Everyman, stricken and stilled, whimpers, 'Death ... I had thee least in mind...'

That's what it's like, the transition. Quite sudden.

Mrs Connely standing with her hand on the door handle with this shadowed look I've seen before, crossing her face. I hear an echo from somewhere past: that always sudden voice interrupting, 'Everyman stand still! Where goest thou so merrily!'

She looked at me, with this odd, other-world expression on her face, and said, 'By the way, Doctor, I meant to mention something...'

That's what it's like – the transition. A beat, nothing more. That first step in the journey that leads from one world to the next.

I pause. I'm running late. I have already mentally closed the file on what was already a pretty congested consultation. But I have been caught before this way. I know that when people say 'By the way…' what they mean is 'this is the thing that matters to me most: the rest was noise.' So I make some time.

I stretch out my hand to indicate the chair she has just now left.

'Sit down.'

It's been going on for about six weeks. At first she thought that it was nothing, then she thought that it was anxiety about her daughter, and now she knows that it's none of these things. A sense at first described as 'fullness', unable to eat very much, gradually morphing into a fluttering, a squeezing, an actual pain. Just an ache, 'a popping feeling, like toothache', not even enough to stop her going to the gym three times a week, but in the middle of the night that ache expands to fill the available mental space: it becomes her whole world. She's always in and out of the toilet, thinking that it will make a difference, but it doesn't, and she might have lost a little weight as well, a pound or two.

Her face goes grey when she climbs onto the scales and sees the evidence of what she's *actually* lost. It is as if she has hopped over some kind of threshold. A step, no more, but she looks thinner to my eye too, now that I know. She climbs briskly onto my couch, eyes a little downcast, all the chatter gone from her. I start with her hands as I always do, then her pulse, the whites of her eyes, looking for jaundice, and other things, and then make my way to her stomach, asking her to pull her gym slacks down a little, lift her fleece. There's a fullness about her lower abdomen that isn't fat, and when I put my hands on it she pulls in her breath sharply. She's clearly in a lot of pain. She has a craggy mass in her lower abdomen: hard, unyielding, about the size of a 16-week pregnancy. She has known about this for *weeks,* shared it with no one. I let her dress. I indicate the chair again. 'Sit down,' I say.

How often does this kind of thing occur? No more than about once every year. But it always still comes as a surprise to me how sudden it is when it happens.

———

Things move very quickly for Mrs Connely. I order her an ultrasound scan of her pelvis, check some bloods.

Generally speaking, in the NHS in my part of Scotland, if a doctor really wants to get something done, and can explain clearly why, provided you make phone calls and are prepared to shepherd your patient through at every step of the way, then things will go quickly and well enough. If you don't, if it's one of the countless other cases that don't seem to you to matter quite so much, then it's as if the system senses it, and your patients can seem to just get lost.

I phone the scan department. I tell them that I think that Mrs Connely probably has an ovarian cancer, and ask them if they can scan her that afternoon. I like Mrs Connely, and her husband, and their troubled daughter. I just can't have them sitting alone at home, wondering, waiting, tortured by uncertainty, by the endless hollow ticking of the old clock they have, standing in their parlour. I can't have this for people I know well, these people who *trust* me.

There's an obvious, lurking injustice here. It has no real defence. I can't care this much about *everyone*. But I am pleased for what I have done, despite whichever unknown other person it is that has been jumped in the scan queue by Mrs Connely, because Mrs Connely's scan is as bad as it could be. It is exactly as I had feared, and I think it's best we know:

An extensive, mainly solid mass in the pelvis, probably arising from ovary, invading other structures, including bladder and bowel, with free pelvic fluid, peritoneal nodules and a suspicion of metastatic disease in the liver...

This is how these kinds of report read.

Because I have been one step ahead throughout this process (I am so often not) I have already arranged an appointment later that week for Mrs Connely at the gynaecology-oncology joint clinic. I don't know if this is any comfort for them, but it is a comfort to me. As I tell them what it is that I have to tell them, I have something at the end to offer. Perhaps it's no more than an empty promise, or an illusion – it's just a *process* after all – but it feels like safe ground. I tell them that there is a structure, a system, a multi-disciplinary team set up to deal with precisely this particular kind of problem: as if the kind of problem she faces is one that can be *dealt with*.

Mrs Connely is a retired art teacher. She is a fan of the Scottish painter John Bellany. She once sent me a thank you card, a copy of a famous portrait of Bellany's grandmother on her death bed: a thin, almost shrivelled woman sitting alone, looking up from her grey sheets gazing imploringly into the face of the painter/ the viewer. There is history etched on the face of that old fisher woman: generations of suffering. You can almost sense the smell of the sick room rising from the canvas. She'd sent me the card as I had seen daughter Annie at short notice, fitted her in, during an emotional crisis. I hadn't really done anything for her, other than listen, but Mrs Connely was grateful to me and wanted to show it. The greeting card was a kind of dark joke between us: understood, but hard to explain. *Thus was our suffering for our daughter: something you could understand.* Today, Mrs Connely has shrunk into herself. Her face is lined and grey. She reeks of pain. She looks up at me, imploringly. Her husband, strong, cut from granite, holds her hand.

Forty-eight hours ago, the pain had seemed a quite peripheral thing. She had been on her way to the gym when she came to see me. She mentioned this pain in passing, an afterthought. It was like a 'popping' sensation, no more. She had almost left without telling me what really ailed her. The transition has changed all of that. The knowledge of the fact that she has crossed from the world of the well to that of the sick has changed her perception of things entirely. The pain now fills her every available space. She sits looking up at me, like Bellany's grandmother, imploring, her hand flat on her lower abdomen, every movement causing her to wince. Forty-eight hours ago, she climbed onto my couch. I wouldn't ask her to do that now.

'How bad is the pain?'

'What do you mean, "how bad"?'

Mrs Connely has never been irritated with me before.

'What is it like?'

'It gnaws away.'

As if a pain might have teeth. For a moment, I feel a scratching low in my stomach. I sense these teeth.

'If I were to ask you to rate it on a scale of one to 10 where one is barely there and 10 is the worst that you could ever imagine, how would you then rate it?'

She ponders.

'When I am busy, when I'm doing things, or before I knew I was sick, it was maybe one, or two. But when I'm thinking about it – like now – or at night, when I'm trying to sleep…'

she winces again, and the power of her body language, subtle as it is, her hand on her stomach, the quiet manner in which she avoids any unnecessary movement, the grey pallor of her once sun-browned skin, communicates something to me, making it all but unbearable to share her space.

'When there is nothing else to think about, it's awful. It's like a six, or even a seven…'

'Seven?'

'Can you please give her something? For her pain?' asks Mr Connely, impatient.

'Of course I will.'

———

I distrust pain measuring scales.

Choose a number on a scale from one to 10, one being barely present, 10 being the worst that you can imagine, to rate your pain.

Choose a face from the frowning one on the left through to the smiley on the right. Which best represents you?

Select a word from this list: *punishing, gruelling, cruel, vicious, killing.* Mark it on the line drawing of a body on the right, and give it a number from one to 20.

People are at their most imaginative and revealing in the words and metaphors that they choose to describe their pain. Consciously or unconsciously, they use every modality of word, language, voice, tone, metaphor, expression, gesture, colour, action, performance and report that is available to them. Educated or not, people become artists, masters of self expression when it comes to the communication of this urgent thing: *I'm in pain.*

The choices that they can make depend on those that are available to them. The pain that comes from pressure on a nerve, for example, what is called 'neuropathic pain', is described, almost always, as 'like an electric shock'. Patients will volunteer that; their physicians will suggest it to them. It's unclear to me what comes first, but when you use the words 'does it feel like an electric shock?' with a person with sciatica, their face will light up with relief, as if they feel at last that their pain is recognised. 'That's it!' they say, 'Like an electric shock!' The metaphor is mutually recognisable: the patient feels understood, and the physician has, fleetingly, a sense of what this suffering might be like if it were theirs. We can all imagine what that must be like: a live wire trailing from the spine, running the length of the nerve, all the way to the feet, discharging periodically, tingling, jolting, searing, burning, like an electric shock. Of course, before electricity, before the 20th century, this metaphor had no shared ground. Then, they used others. Then, neuropathic pain was 'scalding', at a time when everyone knew what it was to be scalded. Or 'like lightning'. Or 'lancinating', at a time when a person might understand what that was, how it felt, to be *lanced*. In the 19th century, pain was often described to doctors as 'furry'. I have no mental impression of what a 'furry' pain might be like. I wonder whether it is the word that has changed, or the pain, or both.

The word 'gout', used for the well-known medical condition, comes from the French word 'gouttelette' to mean a droplet. In Spanish it's 'gota'. It alludes to drops of molten lead splashing on the skin: the metaphor communicating vividly the common understanding shared then by the doctor and his patient, but not shared now, of how a drop of molten lead splashed on the last joint of the big toe would *feel*. 'Gout' is a word and metaphor that has lost its ground.

The words and metaphors that are used to describe pain allow people to share in their subjectivity as best they can. If you don't share a language though, or certain cultural assumptions, or if you lack a certain emotional or empathetic connection, you lose much of the ground that makes this sharing of subjective experience possible. If you don't share a common ground, you are reduced to interpreting gesture, expression, grunts, noises, which is hard. It cuts you off from a person. You begin to doubt. You begin to ask yourself questions like *How much of this is 'real' pain, and how much is just emotion? Or Is this person making it up? For gain? Is this person even capable of pain? Does it really matter?* Or worse: it becomes possible, easy, in fact, to deny the reality, or the validity of your patient's pain, to minimise it, or dismiss it as theatrics, or to treat your patient as somewhat less than human, or at least, less than you. Grunts, noises, cries, moans and screams become wearing after a while, even for the best. Think of a baby on a hot day, on a long train journey, in a crowded, airless carriage, screaming and screaming.

Doctors, in common with just about everyone else, have been rather poor at understanding the reality and validity of the inner lives of people who are even just a little different from them. (When we are hungry, tired, uncomfortable, stressed, frightened, angry, or prejudiced, it makes us even worse.) A list of examples is easy to generate:

+ People from a different culture or who speak a different language;
+ People who look different;
+ People from a different generation;
+ People who are physically or intellectually disabled, or, for whatever reason, can't stand up for themselves;

+ People with a different sexual preference;
+ People with a different, or non-standard, or harder to classify, gender;
+ Slaves – of this, or any era;
+ People from a different social class, or those who have fewer (or more) material possessions;
+ People whom we disapprove of, especially if they are imprisoned.

At their best, pain scales are a way of trying to compensate for this almost universal tendency to undervalue, and undertreat those whom we see as other. Pain scales, now widely and badly used, started as an attempt to create a universal, objective and baggage-free tool for the assessment of pain. But it's not so rare now, that, when I ask a person to describe their pain, they will respond with 'It's a 10!' That doesn't communicate anything to me about that person's pain, other than that they think that it's bad, or that they want me to think that it's bad. Deprived of all of these cultural tools: of language, metaphor, gesture and performance, I feel as if I'm back where I started.

'What exactly do you mean by that? By a … 10?'

I remember lying in a hospital bed once, late at night, with a broken leg, my whole world filled with constant, undertreated pain. I was trying to attract the attention of the preoccupied and busy junior doctor as she hurried by, who kept on avoiding my eye. I think she was tired, over-worked and angry. I think she had me down as a middle-aged drug-seeking wimp who just wanted some attention and needed to 'man up' and go to sleep. (Having been in her shoes myself often enough, I could read her mind effortlessly.)

I wanted to shout out to her 'It's a *10*! *My* pain! It's a *10*!' but she just wasn't listening. I was lonely and scared and I wanted more morphine. I wanted blue lights to flash, and a siren to go off, waking and deafening the whole hospital. My pain was *definitely* a 10.

'It's a 10, Doctor,' says Moira. 'It's *always* an effing 10.'

'What exactly do you mean by that? By ... umm ... 10?'

Moira Bonnet is a rapidly ageing 52. When I call her from the waiting room, she says 'Oof', and struggles slowly to stand, takes an age to organise her sticks, and her bags. I have the feeling that she's making a point. Moira once trusted me; now I think she sees me as the enemy. She walks slowly down the corridor: a slightly waddling gait. She's gaining weight, and I can tell by the way that she uses her hands to help her stand that she has lost muscle in her legs. I stop halfway to my room, waiting for her to catch up. I say something nice about the weather, but she doesn't hear me: she's focusing on her feet. She says, a little irritated, 'I'm just coming,' assuming, I think, that I was trying to hurry her along.

'Ooof.' She whumps down into the chair.

'So much for trying to cut down the tablets,' is her opening.

She catches her breath. She pulls herself up with her stick to sit more upright, holds the posture a moment, then slumps back. She looks tired. She looks at me through thick, blue tinted glasses. Her eyes look melted.

'So ... how is it?'

Always a 10.

There was a husband once, an age ago, but he was an alcoholic, and she kicked him out, but not before he'd drunk their savings. She'd worked in a nursery, and she'd been good at it: she was proud of her work, and all the love that she'd brought to it, but she had to give that up, to look after her father, a whippet thin, demanding old man with a belt and a temper and a tumour on the bowel, who had moderately severe dementia, and died of a haemorrhage, not a moment too soon. She was in receipt of a care allowance, for her father, and now for herself, because she'd developed back pain over the years, from lifting infants, then him. The money doesn't quite compensate for her lost earnings, but she thinks she can't work now whatever.

She was given a prescription in the pain clinic for a strong opiate, and bit by bit the dose has edged up. She is also taking antidepressants, and an anticonvulsant called pregabalin, frequently prescribed for longstanding, non-specific chronic pain, though not licensed for this, and with no good evidence to support its use. The combination, though common, is a trap.

X-rays, scans and bloods repeated every few years, show nothing: a little wear, nothing more and normal for her age. When I remind her of this, she feels it as an assault. Every few months I make it my business to examine her physically: a simple screening test that takes about two minutes and checks every joint in her body, more or less, and it's always normal. She touches her toes, she squats, she duck-walks; she's fine.

'What I don't understand,' she says, angry with me, as she often is, 'is what's actually wrong with me? Is it arthritis like the scan says? Or is it this fibromyalgia, like the achey joint specialist says? Or is it chronic pain like the pain person says? Or is it all in my head? Like you seem to be saying? Or do you all just not have an effing clue?'

When a person answers '10', it can be hard to do anything other than increase the dose, particularly if the doctor's feeling tired, or angry, or stressed, or any of these other things. It's always easier to start a tablet than to stop it, and '10' in this context has come to mean 'give me more,' or 'whatever it is that you're doing, it's not enough.'

Moira's in a kind of medical cul-de-sac. It's common enough. I want to reverse her out of it: my mission is to simplify, reduce, stop.

'Why don't you just take one tablet, at night, to help with sleep. Stop the others. See if you can manage through the day.'

'But what do I do if I have pain…?'

Moira always had that sadness, or so it seemed to me. She was always slow in her movement, weighed down more heavily by gravity. She always moved as if through a denser substance than air. She would say if I asked, and I have asked her many times, that without the heavy drugs she takes, she'd be *finished*. She might be right: who would know better than she? But I think also, the opiate has summoned something from within her: fed it, grown it, made it so that these qualities are all she is now, with hardly anything else besides remaining. It can often seem that way with these drugs, that they bring out something shadowy, empty, ravenous, from deep inside.

———

But what do you *really* think ails Moira?
I don't know…
Yes you do. Go on. What do you *really* think?
Really?
Really.
I think, at bottom, she's lonely. I think she's crushed by loneliness.
And does morphine work for that? Loneliness?

I have never seen it work.

Then why do you prescribe it?

When I next see her, Mrs Connely is quite changed. Mrs Connely seems almost energised by the challenges that she faces. Mr Connely's eyes, however, are bright with this morning's tears. His skin sags from his face. He is almost silent.

In couples who have loved one another for a long time, it can seem as if the membrane that separates one soul from the other has become thinned and permeable, so that suffering seeps between them. One takes the other's load, emotional tasks become divided, sometimes unexpectedly. Mr Connely is already started on the hard work of grieving. I suspect that he is drinking too much. I'm worried for him, even now. Mrs Connely, on the other hand, is slightly buzzy – she has problems to solve.

'Doctor, if you were in my shoes, what questions would you be asking the oncologist?'

She has already had her first clinic appointment. The gynaecologist was kind, she took all the time she needed, but the answers seem clear, even this early. There wasn't any curative surgical option, things were too advanced. That can sometimes happen with ovarian cancer: the tumour can grow considerably before causing symptoms – they are often picked up late. In this case it's no one's fault, she shouldn't feel bad, though people often do. She thinks that they are going to perform another, more detailed scan, an MRI, to define whether surgery might delay things, and to clarify other therapeutic options, probably chemotherapy. She has glossy black hair, Mrs Connely. She is clearly proud of her hair. She maintains it well, dyes it, I'm sure, though never perceptibly as there are never any roots. She runs strands of her hair between her fingers, an unconscious habit: her anguished, fidgety hands speaking for her: 'I don't want to lose my hair.'

'I don't know. But I know what *I* would ask *you* if I were your oncologist.'

She leans forward, interested. Mr Connely, sensing what's coming, turns half away.

'I would want to know, first of all, whether you had understood your situation…'

'Bad…!' she interrupts, with a grim smile, establishing a point about herself. She understands. Mr Connely, out of her line of sight, flinches, as if he has been struck.

'… and whether you understood the diagnosis, any treatment options, what *could* be achieved…'

She says nothing to this.

'Then I would want to know a lot about what matters to you. What you want from life.' I cast around for the words to say *whatever life is left* – but fail. It seems too early in her journey to say that.

Mr Connely interrupts. 'She has a project … our granddaughter, Kira…' but Mrs Connely silences him with a glance.

'And then I would want to get a sense from you of what you would be prepared to give up to realise those things that matter to you…'

'I don't want to have to wear a bag…' she says, a hand on her stomach, voicing this common fear.

'… and I would want to know what you were frightened of, I'd want to get that out into the open too.'

'I have this … thing … I'm doing with Kira. It's silly…'

'It's not silly…' says Mr Connely, tears now pooling in the great bags under his eyes. Every word that's uttered seems to age him by another year.

'... I had this idea ever since she could hold a pencil ... she and I ... we're doing sea birds, we were going to do all the sea birds in Scotland. Pencils for Kira, watercolours for me. I thought that it was going to take us 20 years ... but maybe in a year ... or six months...'

Something fundamental has changed. Something has moved on. This is exactly the conversation that I should be having with Mrs C. *What has changed?* I don't know. I should try asking her about her pain.

'How's your pain?'

That, after all, had been my main reason for seeing her again so soon. I'd actually forgotten. Faced with this urgency – uncontrolled pain consuming a woman I knew (and liked), a young woman with this new, sinister diagnosis – I had gone from a standing start to a prescription for very strong opiates in one step. That always feels risky to me: I'm a little frightened of opiates – opiate-phobic, as it is said. I felt the need to follow her up.

But Mrs Connely just looks at me, frowning, as if to ask 'what pain?' Then, remembering, suppressing a shudder, looking inwardly, deep for an instant in introspective thought, says as if it doesn't matter – and it doesn't, not any more – 'A one...' then frowns a little, '... perhaps a two, when I think about it...'

Just three days prior, I had started her on a tiny dose of sustained release morphine, and a sixth of that for 'breakthrough pain'. Something for her guts, something to stop her from being sick. Almost nothing. These drugs can be so powerful, so good, so easy to prescribe.

'... but that's been really helpful, that *chat*,' she says, changing the subject back again to what really matters. 'I need to remember all that. What matters to me: time with Kira. Watercolours.'

'Hold that thought,' I say.

Mr Connely breaks a smile.

———

Freed from pain, Mrs Connely is able to set her mind now to these urgent life and death questions: what is important, now that time seems short? What *matters* to me? And what would I give up for that? What am I most frightened of? What's my bottom line? What would be unacceptable to me? I can scarcely think of a better use of medical time and skill. I can scarcely think of a better use of medical technology, of drugs: to free a person up to ask that important question 'what *matters* to me, now that life seems short?' If medicine has a purpose, it seems to me, then this must be near to its core.

The fact that I can even think in this way situates me in a particular time and place in culture. We are secular in our outlook, Mrs Connely and I, and that affects how we interpret pain, and what it means to us. It hasn't always been like that. Neither Mrs Connely nor I see her pain as anything other than a harm – a thing she needs to be unshackled from, if she is to be restored to herself, to see the world right again. Mrs Connely, she and I believe, has a right to be free of her pain – or at least a right to be given every assistance to be free of her pain. We don't see her pain as a kind of spiritual learning opportunity. We don't see it as a test. We don't see her pain as the consequence of anybody's sin, and we don't see her suffering of her pain as necessary for the expiation of that sin. We don't think that her pain will ennoble her, nor buy her, or others, time free from punishment, nor do we see it as a gift from God, to enable her to focus her mind on salvation, and we don't see in its treatment, a risk to her eternal soul. Mrs Connely doesn't see in her pain an opportunity to emulate the sufferings of Christ, and I don't see in her pain the opportunity to teach her about her own vanities and shortcomings in faith. In fact it seems completely outlandish to me that anyone might ever harbour such ideas. Archaic, barbaric even. No one, now, thinks like that. Although doctors, their patients and their ministers and priests had wrestled seriously with these worries for centuries, we've left these problems behind us. They don't affect us in any way whatsoever, now, or at least we don't think that they do. But people in pain are always *social beings* in pain: the way that they experience their pain, how they understand it, what it means, how it *feels*, depends on their history, their culture and their beliefs. We may not know explicitly what these are, we may be quite unaware that they exist, but we can't escape them.

People have known about the effects of morphine for 200 years, opium for centuries, but something has stopped us from using them. Barriers to the use of opiates are multiple and deeply ingrained. People worry about addiction. People have an image in their head of a broken, beseeching drug addict, deprived of his personhood, despised in his community. Old people, sick people, on the very edge of death, needing help to die, ask 'will these drugs make me into an addict?' People fear that starting strong opiates has the effect of confirming their dismal prognosis. By taking effective steps to control their pain, they are making it *real*. They remember their own relative, late and deep into their illness, how, so shortly after the nurse first administered morphine, they slipped far into themselves, lost their contact with the world, fell insensible, and died. People can confuse causes and effects, the natural order of things.

Doctors, underskilled in their use, worry about killing people with opiates. When I was a new trainee in general practice, I was called to an old woman's house. A churchy lady in a tartan skirt, she had a sudden onset of heart failure and was drowning in lung fluids. The standard treatment in hospital for this, back then, was intravenous heroin, which gives almost immediate relief to breathlessness and distress. In hospital, they also have readily available oxygen and resuscitation equipment. She fell like a tree with the modest dose that I gave her and the ambulance technicians had to let themselves into her house, because I couldn't abandon the artificial respiration that I was engaged in for long enough to let them in. She was fine in the end. She sent me a thank you card. I was less fine. It created a barrier in me, a caution when starting elderly people on opiates, that I might inadvertently harm them, or even kill.

Legal controls around the use of strong opiates haven't helped. The disaster of the Harold Shipman case means that GPs now, by and large, no longer carry strong opiates in their bags. Most of the time that's not a problem, help being generally close to hand. Sometimes, though, it's catastrophic.

Patients and their doctors value stoicism. People don't want to be a burden, they don't want to seem to be weak, or moaning, or dull. Doctors favour untroublesome patients: they like the quiet, uncomplaining, grateful, undemanding types, the ones that do *well*, and get *better*. These values have deep roots. It's not just doctors who are like this – families are, too. With pain, sometimes, you have to ask, again and again, before people will admit to it, and sometimes they never do. I have known patients die what *I* had thought to be a good death, well managed, and their relatives, after, reflecting, will tell me how grateful they are, how well it all went, until the end, of course, when the suffering grew terrible … And I hadn't known. Although I had asked, over and over, I still hadn't known. People – patients, their families, their doctors – often think that there is something inevitable, *normal*, acceptable, about suffering at the end of life.

Attitudes to pain management in terminal care changed profoundly with the hospice movement. Hospice care has always been one step outside mainstream medical practice in the UK. It retains a ghost of its religious origins: more than is usual in modern medicine, at least. It concerns itself more with *spirit* and *soul*, without using these words. The movement distinguishes clearly between duration of life, and its purpose. It seems more open-minded, more flexible, patient-centred and holistic in its outlook.

Hospices are practical too: they deal with things like housing and benefits entitlements, if money or housing is where the problem is. They are accessible. I have the number for Mrs Connely's two hospice nurses on my mobile phone. We are on first name terms. We have collaborated in the management of dying patients for years. When things go wrong, they call me directly, or I call them, and they recognise my voice on the phone.

The hospice movement helps opiate-afraid doctors with evidence: clear and concise, easily available guidelines for the management of cancer symptoms. A treatment ladder, which escalates, rung by rung, from paracetamol and aspirin at the bottom, to strong opiates like morphine or oxycodone at the top. Clear rules for the diagnosis of kinds and causes of pain; clear strategies and colour coded checklists to guide us in the management of each.

Doctors and nurses, the more experienced they get – the more specialised, and the more exposed to it – the *worse* they tend to get at estimating the pain's severity. They grow thick skins – perhaps they have to. Hospice nurses challenge our pain insensitivity, and have been leaders in the promotion of object-ive pain-rating scales to combat it. That's why we use these pain-rating scales – why we ask these facile 'rate it on a scale of one to 10' questions – to pare away this horny leather shell we all seem to grow to protect our sensitive inner parts. And this revolutionary ideology has, slowly, slowly, bled into the rest of medical culture. More and more, the idea that doctors, nurses, dentists, expect their patients to just put up with pain is intoler-able. People have a *right* to be free of pain, and their doctors have an absolute duty to recognise it. And quite right too.

But the sweetest of dreams can curdle.

I met Lyra Trembath first about a month ago. A refugee, from Cornwall. She is six inches taller than I am, a well-worn forty-something with unkempt hair and teeth, ranging arms and broken nails. She wears skinny jeans with a huge ornate buckle and a long striped smock, and uses a stick when she walks, with a knobbled end carved like a skull. When she sits she folds into herself like an old-style wooden deck chair.

She is newly registered with us: a temporary resident in a hostel, fled from a violent relationship at home, she has moved from place to place to escape her stalking, controlling man, and she has washed up here. She will be with us for a month or two, a year at most, and then she will move on. We have a number of women on our list like this, like Lyra, internal refugees from domestic war, always on the move. Their needs are often over-whelming. We never get to know them well, never have the time to even begin to make a difference, and then they're gone.

'I'm just here for my prescription, Doctor.'

She has a friendly and open manner. She has a strong West Country accent which I almost never get to hear; she has a sweet, witchy, snaggle-toothed smile.

'What's that then?'

'The pill.'

Easy enough.

'And them…'

She passes me an empty blister pack and a packet with a barely legible label: 'Oxycontin 40mg, twice daily.'

That's much harder. Practically the strongest opiate there is. That would be a lethal dose, for you or me.

'How long have you been taking these?'

'My last doctor gave them to me. He wanted to put up the dose.'

'What are they for?'

'My back pain. I think. I think he said they were for my back pain…'

'Do they help?'

'I … think so…'

'Are you taking anything else for your pain?'

'These … and these … and these …,' she says, passing me more empty packets with names I cannot even read.

'I've run out. My last doctor warned me not to stop them suddenly.'

Quite right. Everyone knows what happens if you stop taking high doses of opiates, suddenly. Anxiety, agitation, insomnia, gooseflesh, sweating, bone-breaking cramps, diarrhoea, constipation, headaches, all over body pain, vomiting, fits, delirium, inhalation pneumonia, sometimes death.

'When did you run out?'

'At the weekend.'

It's already Tuesday afternoon.

'How are you feeling?'

'A bit tired. I've not been sleeping very well. There's a lot of noise in the hostel. Lots of screaming. I was actually wondering if you could give me a letter for the housing...'

'How's your back pain?'

'That's just the same. Nothing really makes much difference to that...'

When I examine her, her knees click. Her back creaks like an old hinge: she folds herself in two like a step ladder, the palms of her two hands laid flat on the floor, crooked bony fingers tapered, like two spider crabs. She straightens up, a little out of breath, but there is grace and elegance still in how she packs this awkward body of hers. She doesn't *seem* to be in any pain.

'Has anybody told you why you have back pain?'

'My last doctor said that I have arthritis of the spine. A specialist told me I've got hypermobility ... I don't know what I've got!'

I nod. This combination of vague diagnosis and lethal drug combination is commoner in modern medical practice than you might think. We build ourselves traps that can be hard to escape. Not today, as it happens.

I ask her: 'Do you *want* to be on all these drugs?'

She says, 'No ... of course not...' *Stupid question.* 'But my last doctor told me not to stop them suddenly. Is there a problem with them?'

There is an enormous problem, in my view. In fact, three enormous problems:

1   The one thing that we know for sure about the management of non-specific chronic pain is that it responds to gradual physical rehabilitation: to exercise, to

movement, to being out in the world, walking the dog, doing your shopping, climbing the stairs, going to the park with your children, kicking a ball around with your chums, going to the gym, whatever it is that lights your fire. And the one consistent effect of being on high strength opiates is that it stops you from doing any of these things.

2 There is nothing more miserable than being in constant pain. Everything that you do to manage your pain needs to help you to manage your mood at the same time. But to be on long term opiates is to live life in the shade. They make you gloomy and depressed.

3 They don't work. After the initial kick, the euphoria, the dizzying glee resulting from being rendered indifferent to the pain that's eating you, they leave you in a few weeks pretty much as you were before, until the next dose increase, at least. But they also leave you vulnerable: to lethargy, confusion, falls, drug interactions, overdoses, depression, dementia, weight gain, pneumonia, muscle loss, addiction, theft, constipation, early death.

'So,' I conclude, 'they're not ideal, but…'

'Well I'll just stay off them then! If they're *that* dangerous, I won't take them…'

'No, I mean … Hang on, what I mean…'

'No! I'll stop them!'

'Maybe just reduce them a bit?' I say, back-pedalling, but…

'No way! I'm stopping them!'

I have strong opinions about all this. My colleagues might say, an obsession. Mainly, I keep these feelings to myself, or try, but sometimes they just seep out. I think that we are implicated in a medical and social disaster. I think that we are living through an epidemic of chronic pain and opiate misuse – I think the pain and the opiates feed one another. I think that the medical profession and the pharmaceutical industry have fed both. I think that we are *vectors* in this epidemic. And I think that this epidemic is driven by an ideology: what has been called a 'doxogenic epidemic'. I think this ideology is raised upon the following sturdy pillars:

+ All pain is subjective and equally valid;
+ It can be objectively measured using validated pain scales;
+ It should be assessed and recorded as routinely as any other vital sign: pulse, blood pressure, respiratory rate, temperature;
+ Everyone has a *right* to be pain free.

But pain just isn't like that. There is tissue-damage pain, such as the pain of a broken leg, or post-operative pain, or cancer pain, for example, all of which respond to opiates beautifully. There is chronic, non-specific back-pain which is a complex social and psychological phenomenon, with some physical aspects to it, whose treatment needs to address each of these interacting and difficult-to-resolve aspects. These phenomena are at different ends of a spectrum with a whole lot in between. I don't think that that one word, 'pain', bears the same meaning across this bandwidth.

But it's much easier, time-saving, less philosophically complex, cheaper (in the short term), less adversarial, more validating, less controversial, to ignore all this and to simply prescribe opiates, and then increase them, and then increase them again. They generally make people feel a little better, in the short term, if a little *drugged*. But they undermine, sometimes destroy, the possibility of recovery. And I think that this is the laziest kind of medicine, and we need to be ashamed of ourselves for letting it happen. All of which puts me out on a limb, medically speaking. And being a maverick in medicine is never good.

Having loosened a little the spigot on my opinions with Lyra, I tried to jam it tight back shut again, but I'm too late. She's just *stopped all her drugs*, and any harm that comes to her as a consequence, will be my fault. But I needn't have worried. Lyra comes back to see me a few days later, to pick up her letter for the housing people. I'm pleased to see her – I like her *oddness*, the skull carved on the knobble-end of her stick. Today she reminds me of an umbrella. She's still a little tired. She still complains of the same old pain, but moves smoothly, unfurling those long limbs easily enough. She hands me a packet of paracetamol, asks me whether it's safe to take them. I say yes, safe enough.

An evening visit to Mrs Connely's.

There will come a time, perhaps in just a few weeks, when I will come back to visit this house and it will be silent again.

In a few weeks' time I will come here to find Mr Connely on his own, unslept, hungover, bloated, walking from room to room to empty room, as if he's looking for something that he has lost, footsteps followed by the hollow ticking of the antique grandfather clock which stands, resonant and solitary in the stair well.

Today though, Mrs Connely is home at last from hospital and the place is full of noise. She sits upright in a hospital bed downstairs in the sitting room, a wide picture window giving a view onto the garden she has tended since she and her husband moved here 35 years before. It's late summer, and the last of the roses are just losing their petals. They have set up a slide and a climbing frame on the lawn, and Kira and a friend are running in circles, shouting, climbing the frame, sliding down the slide, climbing up the frame again.

Mrs Connely has had a rubbish time. She had some surgery, to 'debulk' her tumour, but surgery was aborted. She had some chemotherapy, and she lost her hair, but she avoided the colostomy bag that she had feared. Her hair is growing in again, but it's grey and thin, and she keeps it covered now. She has had some hospital admissions with intestinal obstruction, but that seems fixed for now. There was an option for more chemotherapy, but she has declined that: she sees now that she has this brief window of being, relatively speaking, well, and she wants to be home. She fears a constant declining cycle of hospital admissions. Her bottom line is this: she wants to be at home, she wants to see the last of the summer in her garden. She is attached to a syringe driver that delivers a constant dose of opiates and antiemetics. Between myself and Bridget the hospice nurse, we seem to have the dose just right.

I'm chatting to Mrs Connely. I have this facile checklist in my head which I tick off as we talk: pain; drugs; nausea; guts; bladder; pressure sores; nourishment; mood; spirits; soul. I'm chatting to Mrs Connely, while Annie, her daughter, is perched on a stepladder. Annie is hanging mobiles from the ceiling: cut-out birds she's made with Kira with watercolours and crayons: gannets, gulls, puffins, petrels, skua, cormorants, terns. Scottish seabirds. Then Juan comes in, interrupting, bearing armfuls of nursing clutter that the team will need in the days and weeks ahead, he's just picked it all up from the chemist. He sees Annie on the stepladder, and me, standing with my bag, and he greets us both with a smile. Mrs Connely says: 'In the bathroom, Juan! Don't leave them there!' She speaks sharply to him. He doesn't deserve it. But she still hasn't quite forgiven him.

Moira's back to see me.

Everything with Moira is *so* adversarial. *Everything* is an argument. Moira today is aggressively better. She strides down the corridor, practically takes me down as she passes. The sticks are gone. The 'Ooof' is absent. She has slung over her shoulder a canvas bag full of summer stock and freshly cut herbs: there are thyme, chives and a bunch of coriander. When she sits, these medieval scents fill my room, and I think *why don't I keep fresh-cut herbs on my windowsill? Why don't all doctors do that?*

'Well, you were wrong about the tablets, Doctor. Look.'

She stands, stretches, touches her toes, stands, takes a deep breath, adopts the warrior pose, stops, touches her toes, does a sun salutation, stands, takes a deep breath in, smiles, says, 'Couldn't do that before, could I?'

'No…'

'Well I tried what you suggested. I tried stopping the tablets and I was like an old woman! Couldn't even get up the stairs! So I thought *effit* and did what I'd wanted to do all along, started taking one of the tablets in the morning, one of the tablets in the evening, one in the middle of the day if I wanted it, just like you told me *not to*. That was three weeks ago, and for the last three weeks I've been champion!' She flexes her bicep.

'Well … that's … great…,' I say, revising again all my precious, *stupid* theories about pain.

'So I just need another prescription and I won't take up any more of your valuable time.'

'O ... kay...,' I say, turning to the computer. 'What's with the lovely herbs?' I ask, hoping, improbably, that they might be a present for me.

'They're for Mickey.'

'Who's Mickey?'

'He's my new lodger. He lets me share his allotment in exchange for rent. It's great. I knew him from work. He called me three weeks ago because he'd split up with his boyfriend. He just moved straight into dad's old room. We're like an old married couple,' she says, standing now, with her prescription in her hand, heading for the door, '... though without the sex, thank God! I make him breakfast and he does the supper, and in the evening we watch black and white movies and musicals. See you, Doc.'

And what is the cure for the pain of loneliness?

A friend. In the case of loneliness, surely, a friend would be the cure.

NOTES ON SOURCES

THE REAL KARLO PISTAZJA

For the original 17th century account of his *forensic* definition of personhood, try:

Locke, John, *An Essay Concerning Human Understanding*: *Book II: Ideas* (1689) Chapter xxvii, Identity and Diversity.

And for its 20th century dismantling:

Parfit, Derek, 'Personal Identity', *The Philosophical Review* 8(1) (1971), 3–27 http://www.jstor.org/stable/2184309

THE WORDS TO SAY IT

Shorter, Edward, *From Paralysis to Fatigue: A History of Psychosomatic Illness in the Modern Era* (1991), The Free Press

An excellent historical account of how doctors and society have viewed functional disorders, together with thoughts on the physical, social, psychological and cultural origins of these symptoms, can be found in *From Paralysis to Fatigue*. I have borrowed ideas developed by Shorter, debated them with friends and colleagues, and used the results extensively in this book, and, indeed, in my own medical practice, and I am indebted to his work.

Stone, Jon, 'Functional Symptoms in Neurology', *Practical Neurology* 9 (2009), 179-189.

For Dr Marks' account of the different ways in which functional disorders are labelled by doctors, and how these labels are perceived by patients, I have borrowed and adapted from Dr Jon Stone's article.

Stone's website www.neurosymptoms.org is a fantastic resource for patients and their clinicians for both understanding, coping with, and finding the words to talk about, this complex and difficult family of conditions.

SHANGALANG

Gillon, Raanan, 'Medical Ethics: Four Principles Plus Attention to Scope', *British Medical Journal* 16, 309(6948) (1994): 184-188

For a concise and readable account of the 'four principles' approach to thinking about medical ethics, see Gillon's article. Professor Gillon's advocacy of the original work of Beauchamp and Childress has influenced a generation of students and doctors, providing us with a firm platform to be able to think clearly and dispassionately about ethical problems in medicine.

'... *I have never found appeals to God helpful...*'

This is a version of the dilemma posed in Plato's *Euthyphro*: 'Is what is pious loved by the Gods because it is pious, or is it pious because it is loved by the Gods?'

THREE VIEWS OF A MOUNTAIN

Aviv, Rachel, 'The Apathetic', *The New Yorker*, 23/7/17

For 'Resignation Syndrome'.

Hacking, Ian, *Rewriting the Soul: Multiple Personality and the Science of Memory* (1995), Princeton University Press

Hacking, Ian, *Mad Travellers: Reflections on the Reality of Transient Mental Illnesses* (1998), University of Virginia Press

I have borrowed the idea of vectors acting on human behaviour, and how people, when experiencing certain kinds of illness, are obliged to act under those descriptions of illness which are culturally available to them, from the Canadian philosopher Ian Hacking, who describes, in his books, the conditions, or vectors that he sees as being necessary for epidemics of what he calls 'transient mental illness'. Reading Hacking's work transformed my view of the philosophy of medicine: indeed it introduced me to the concept that there might be such a thing. His thinking is clear, engaging, and available to the non-specialist, and I would recommend him to any interested reader.

WHEN DARKNESS FALLS

'*The effect of a classification system that looks biological, is to affect the way that we think about it...*'

This idea is borrowed from the review 'Lost in the Forest', of the *Diagnostic and Statistacal Manual* (V), by Ian Hacking, *London Review of Books*, August 2013

Healy, David, *The Anti-Depressant Era* (1999), Harvard University Press.

For a fascinating and readable account of the history of depression in psychiatry, and the influence of the science of brain chemistry on how we think about mood and how we experience it, try this. I have borrowed extensively from Healy's ideas for this chapter, including the image of the biochemical key fitting a lock whose shape is pre-determined by companies marketing both an illness and a cure.

Borch-Jacobsen, Mikkel, 'Psychotropicana', *London Review of Books*, July 11, 2002

For a briefer and accessible account of the relationship between mood, society, the medical profession and the pharmaceutical industry, try this essay.

Yalom, Irvin D., *Love's Executioner, and Other Tales of Psychotherapy* (1968), Penguin.

'Everything comes to an end….' The austere thoughts and reflections which follow here evolved from the introduction to this book.

THE GHOST IN THE MACHINE

Dennett, Daniel C., 'Why You Can't Make a Computer That Feels Pain.' *Synthese* 38, no. 3 (1978): 415-56. http://www.jstor.org/stable/20115302.

My model of a 'web of interconnecting boxes and lines…' together with my idea of constructing a 'pain machine,' as a way of illustrating the difficulties we have framing exactly what we *mean* by pain, is influenced by the philosopher Daniel Dennett in this essay.

OPIATES ARE THE OPIATE OF THE PEOPLE PT II

Bourke, Joanna, *The Story of Pain: From Prayer to Painkillers* (2014), OUP.

For my reflections on the cultural history of pain and its diverse meanings, I was immensely helped and influenced by Joanna Bourke's book.

Quinones, Sam, *Dreamland* (2015), Bloomsbury.

Lembke, Anna, *Drug Dealer, MD, How Doctors Got Duped, Patients Got Hooked and Why It's So Hard to Stop* (2016), Johns Hopkins University Press.

A great deal has been written about the 'medical disaster' of the epidemic of chronic pain and its relationship with over-treatment by doctors with strong opiates, particularly in the US. Examples include *Dreamland*, which is an excellent, accessible and compelling read, and *Drug Dealer, MD*, which offers a more medical perspective.

ACKNOWLEDGEMENTS

I have been very fortunate in the support that I have received from patients, friends, family, colleagues, and various experts and specialists whom I have consulted in the research and writing of *The Human Kind*.

My partners in practice, Doctors Aileen Telfer and Stuart Blake, have been patient and generous, both with the enormous amounts of time away from my medical duties that they have permitted me, but also with putting up for years with my many obsessions, rants and hobby-horses, which I'm sure must be trying. It's not possible to practise medicine happily, without kind, trusted, critical colleagues watching your back.

Where an individual patient might recognise something of their own self or their story in an account, I have taken care to ask their permission, discussed my intentions with them, and have been deeply grateful for their openness and willing participation. The details and trajectories of the emergent characters have all been altered, and altered again, to make them unidentifiable to a third person.

I would particularly like to mention Mrs J.A. whose kind and intelligent reading of some of my material pointed a way forward for me at a difficult time.

Three Views of a Mountain continues to hang on my wall, and I would like to thank its painter yet again for this gift.

As a child, the adults in our lives give us permission for what we might do or become. I would like to thank my uncle Dr Morrison Dorward for his lifelong example of what compassion, care, and love, lived, might look like.

I was a terrible student and medical trainee, and I would like to thank again those teachers who had the patience and kindness to soldier on with my medical education. In particular, Dr Iain Lamb, to whom I owe a debt for much of what I think is positive in my practice as a generalist, and as a medical teacher. When I speak with doctors who struggle (we all sometimes struggle...), it's his voice that I hear.

When I discovered, late, that medicine has an indispensable ethical and philosophical dimension, it changed my trajectory, and created in me a deep and sustained fascination which has enlivened my career and made me a better doctor. I would like to thank Prof. Raanon Gillon for years of friendship, education, support and fun. His advice has always mattered to me, and it was he who started me out on this journey.

I would have been quite unable to begin to write *The Human Kind* without the friendship of Dr Gavin Francis. He was there right at the beginning of the project, and was the first to read the finished manuscript. I can't thank him enough for his support. Our best friends make us more than we could otherwise be.

I would like to thank Dr Thomas Williams who read and corrected every chapter, who has kept me straight and sane, and whose advice and friendship have sustained me for years. Responsibility for any errors of fact, taste or style in the final work remains his.

Prof. Andrew Canessa has been an unfailing source of friendship and solace for decades – whether one is stuck on a rock face, or stumped by a recipe, his words are always well judged and feedback invaluable. My Jacha Chuymani.

Dr Douglas Dorward helped me more than he knows by listening to me talk and commenting on the material that he kindly read for me.

Mark Halliley offered me detailed comments on chapters at an early stage; his thoughts were spot on, and his support immensely encouraging at a time when I needed it.

Thank you to Sophie Balhetchet whose concise, perceptive editorial advice was hugely valued. Collaborating on projects with Sophie has always been a privilege and a joy.

I would like to thank Ruth Mackenzie again, for her kind encouragement, and for the use of her flat to write: hers has the best view in all Amsterdam.

Andrea Joyce and Andrew Dorward must have read thousands of pages of my work over the years. Every writer needs kind, critical readers, every person needs the love of kind and critical friends – so thank you again for so many years of both.

Frank Wintle has been the greatest of readers and friends. I'm grateful for his time and careful critical feedback. He is also the most joyous holiday/writing/cooking companion a person might ever wish for.

I'm grateful to Dr Lizzie Wastnedge for her reading of several chapters and for her valuable comments and encouragement.

Dr John Dunn is a great teaching colleague and a friend, a brilliant medical educator, and fantastic advocate on behalf of good medicine. I was grateful for the time he took over the material that I asked him to read, and for his perceptive and helpful comments.

Prof. Frank Cogliano is a great host, a wonderful story teller and a good friend. I was encouraged and moved by his kind response to the chapter that I asked him to read.

Thank you also to David Scott for the long walks, good company, and for listening to me talk, and talk, for years.

Several specialists in their fields of medicine and philosophy have been generous with their time, advice and support for *The Human Kind*:

My friend Dr Tim Dalkin was helpful in taking the time to tactfully correct my misunderstandings around schizophrenia and the Mental Health Act. The residual errors and inaccuracies are mine.

Dr Jon Stone was generous with his time, knowledge and advice, and I am grateful to him for both taking my thoughts seriously, and for encouraging me to try them out on his clinical colleagues, whose feedback and comments were gracious and helpful.

Dr Ivan Marples kindly allowed me time and space to discuss with him my thoughts, and was, in hindsight, incredibly tolerant and decent in his response to my criticisms of the medical model for chronic pain and its treatment.

The philosopher in the attic room in Glasgow is Dr David Bain. I am grateful to him for his kind hospitality, for quietly seeing through the nonsense, and then finding and engaging with what was interesting about my argument. His input was enormously encouraging. As I say, every doctor feeling paralysed by the incoherencies in their field should have a generous philosopher with whom to consult.

In my few years of knowing Prof. Tim Engstrom, he has been an enormous source of encouragement and clarity: he has helped me with several chapters and I have valued his broad cultural knowledge and critical responses, as well as enjoying walks, conversation, book recommendations and gracious company.

My agent Jenny Brown at JBA could not have been more receptive, open and helpful, offering support, practical advice and encouragement at exactly those moments when I have needed it.

Charlotte Croft has been an absolute delight to work with in the preparation of *The Human Kind*. I am grateful to her and to all of the staff at Bloomsbury who have been involved in the project, for their engagement, encouragement and trust.

Finally, I would like to thank my partner Deborah, for everything, and our two boys, Jack and Jamie, for helping to make life so precious.